A Natural Approach

Obesity, Weight Loss and Eating Disorders

Macrobiotic Health Education Series

MACROBIOTIC HEALTH EDUCATION SERIES

A Natural Approach

Obesity, Weight Loss and Eating Disorders

by Michio Kushi

edited by John D. Mann

foreword by Lawrence Haruo Kushi, Sc.D.

Japan Publications, Inc.

Tokyo · New York

Note to the reader: Those with health problems are advised to seek the
guidance of a qualified medical, or psychological professional in addition
to that of a qualized macrobiotic courselor before implementing any of the
dietary and other approaches presented in this book. It is essential that any
reader who has any reason to suspect serious illness in themselves or
their family members seek appropriate medical, nutritional, or psychological advice promptly. Neither this or any other health related book
should be used as a substitute for qualified care or treatment.

Published by JAPAN PUBLICATIONS, INC., Tokyo and New York

Distributors:
UNITED STATES: *Kodansha International/USA, Ltd., through Harper & Row,
Publishers, Inc., 10 East 53rd Street, New York, New York 10022.* SOUTH
AMERICA: *Harper & Row, Publishers, Inc., International Department.*
CANADA: *Fitzhenry & Whiteside Ltd., 195 Allstate Parkway, Markham,
Ontario, L3R 4T8.* MEXICO AND CENTRAL AMERICA: *HARLA S. A. de C. V.,
Apartado 30–546, Mexico 4, D. F.* BRITISH ISLES: *International Book Dis-
tributors Ltd., 66 Wood Lane End, Hemel Hempstead, Herts HP2 4RG.*
EUROPEAN CONTINENT: *Fleetbooks, S. A., c/o Feffer and Simons (Nederland)
V. V., Rijnkade 170, 1382 GT Weesp, The Netherlands.* AUSTRALIA AND
NEW ZEALAND: *Bookwise International, 1 Jeanes Street, Beverley, South
Australia 5007.* THE FAR EAST AND JAPAN: *Japan Publications Trading.
Co., Ltd., 1-2-1, Sarugaku-cho, Chiyoda-ku, Tokyo 101.*

First edition: June 1987

LCCC No. 85–081368
ISBN 0–87040–641–8

Printed in U.S.A.

Foreword ━━━━━━━━━━━━━━━━━━━━━━━━━━

This particular volume of the *Macrobiotic Health Education Series* concerns itself with obesity, a condition many nutritionists agree is the major food-related disorder afflicting people in the United States today. Certainly, overweight is a risk factor for the major causes of death and disability. It is a contributor to heart disease, several types of cancer, and diabetes.

If we consider obesity as one extreme on a spectrum of eating disorders, then anorexia nervosa and bulimia are, in the United States, the other extreme. Yet, as is so often the case, the two extremes are often products of similar circumstance. Thus, we come to appreciate the paradox that results in anorexia and bulimia reaching epidemic proportion in our society, while at the same time overweight is a major physical and social problem.

It is generally recognized that there are two major factors that contribute to obesity in the United States. The first is the increasingly sedentary lifestyle to which we have adapted over the past several decades. This is easily appreciated by realizing that we rely on microwave ovens to heat our pre-packaged meals; our automobiles take us from our front door to our work place; and we ride elevators and escalators instead of using the stairs. Many of us must make a concerted effort to physically challenge ourselves by scheduling time at the local fitness club. Contrast this lifestyle with that experienced by most of our grandparents and great-grandparents, who probably were farmers or could at least relate closely to gardening and agriculture, and who probably engaged in more physical activity in their daily lives than we can manage to schedule into ours. Thus, even though we are eating less per capita now than we did at the turn of the century, we also weigh more.

The other major factor that contributes to obesity in our society is the excess fat in the diet of most Americans. It is the nature of foodstuffs that, gram for gram, fat contains more energy than either protein or carbohydrate. It is no surprise, then, that other things being equal, a high-fat diet leads to consumption of more calories and the need to store more calories in the form of body fat.

At the same time that we are faced with a diet that promotes weight gain and a lifestyle that discourages weight loss, we are confronted with societal ideals of body shape that promote slimmer figures than was the ideal several decades ago. Not surprisingly, we are forced into a situation where extreme attempts to attain ideal body shapes turn into potentially devastating eating disorders.

Readers of this book will gain an understanding of the origins of these disorders, and will be introduced to guidelines for preventing and dealing with them. Additional insights include an appreciation for the natural order of our bodies and the health-promoting vigor of regular physical activity, along with a broader perspective on personal and social images of body shape. The insights one can gain from this book, along with the practicle suggestions found in the companion cookbook, can lead to a healthier spirit, mind, and body.

Lawrence Haruo Kushi, Sc.D.
Minneapolis, Minnesota
December, 1986

Introduction

One of the glaring results of the modern diet and lifestyle is the problem of overweight. The overconsumption of saturated fat, sugar, refined flour, and processed food, combined with a lack of exercise and physical activity, has led to this epidemic.

The accumulation of fat in the body sets the stage for a variety of problems. When fat clogs the arteries, the result is heart disease. When it lines the intestine, the absorption of nutrients is diminished, and the result may be malnutrition. Fat clogging the kidneys leads to improper filtering of the blood.

The extremes in diet so common today—when combined with psychological and social stress—can create a variety of eating disorders, of which *bulimia*, or the "binge-purge" syndrome, and *anorexia nervosa*, or the compulsive refusal to eat, are examples.

Although psychological factors play a role in these conditions, the underlying cause can be found in the imbalances inherent in the modern way of eating and way of life.

Today, millions of people are seeking solutions to the problem of weight control by following various fad diets. Yet, because such approaches are often unbalanced or extreme, individuals are unable to loose weight satisfactorily or to achieve good health. For many people, the world "diet" has negative connotations such as restricting oneself to a narrow range of foods or limiting intake by fasting or skipping meals.

Unlike restrictive approaches, the macrobiotic way of life offers a practically unlimited range of foods, combinations, and cooking methods. And, unlike fad diets, macrobiotics is based on humanity's traditional dietary patterns. Macrobiotics allows one to avoid many of the potentially harmful elements in the modern diet, while enjoying an incredibly wide range of whole natural foods.

Hundreds of thousands of people around the world have achieved optimum weight and health through the macrobiotic way of life. People who practice macrobiotics are generally noted for their trim, healthy figures; with the kind of physiques that are associated with reduced rates of degenerative illness and an improved quality of life.

The dietary guidelines presented in this book are consistent with similiar recommendations for disease prevention made by leading public health agencies, including the U.S. Senate Committee on Nutrition and Human Needs, the American Cancer Society, the American Heart Association, and the National Academy of Sciences. A low fat, high fiber diet based around complex carbohydrates—such as those found in whole cereal grains, fresh local vegetables, beans, and other whole natural foods—is increasingly being recognized as an optimum way of eating for overall health.

Over the past thirty-five years, macrobiotic education has challenged the leading health problems of our century, including cancer, heart disease, diabetes, and recently, AIDS and immune deficiencies. Many macrobiotic suggestions have been adopted by scientific and medical organizations as a part of a developing consensus that diet is a major factor in health and sickness.

This book in the *Macrobiotic Health Education Series* is the first of our publications to address the issue of weight loss in detail. We hope that all those experiencing weight problems or eating disorders can benefit from the simple guidelines and suggestions presented here.

I thank all of our friends who helped in the production of this volume, including our associate John David Mann for compiling and editing the material. I thank Jay Kelly for contributing the artwork, and our associate, Edward Esko, for his guidance and advice in planning and completing the book. I thank my son, Lawrence Haruo Kushi, for writing the Foreword. I extend my deepest appreciation to my wife, Aveline, who, together with our associate, Helaine Honig, completed the companion cookbook in the *Macrobiotic Food and Cooking Series*. I thank our friends, Iwao Yoshizaki and Yoshiro Fujiwara, respectively president and American representitive of Japan Publications, Inc., for their continuing guidance and inspiration. Finally, I thank our associate, Phillip Jannetta, in Tokyo, for doing the editorial work on this book.

Michio Kushi
Brookline, Massachusetts
April, 1987

Contents

10

1. Why Are We Overweight?

Over the past ten years there has been an explosion of scientific studies on the cause and cure of weight problems.[1] This flurry of research is partly fueled by hopes of stemming the endemic tide of obesity's associated health problems, such as heart disease, diabetes, and certain types of cancer. This is especially true since the mid-1970s, when the scientific mainstream and popular press began to broadly acknowledge the importance of diet as a major factor in both the cause and prevention of our leading degenerative diseases. In part, it is also a response to the barrage of ill-informed "quick-weight-loss" schemes and pat answers flooding the mass-media markets.

Concern with obesity in the face of abundance is hardly a new problem in human society. Socrates danced every morning to keep slim; evidently his most famous student did not. Plato's renowned fatness, normally a serious defect in the eyes of the ancient Greeks, was forgiven only on account of his intellectual brilliance.[2] Since the dawn of Western medicine, problems with weight have been routinely observed, pondered and treated as a threat to human health. But in no epoch until the present has overweight risen so dramatically to the swollen prevalence experienced today.

Unfortunately, the recent intensification of research has yielded little in the way of practical results. Researchers have brought to light many of the mechanisms that may be involved in weight control and eating disorders. But nearly all this new knowledge is still hypothetical, and much of it controversial. There is very little consensus on what is actually going on in the body and mind of a person whose weight is out of control. There is even less agreement as to the root cause of such problems, or as to the best courses of treatment.

For example, a much-touted National Institutes of Health (N.I.H.) conference in February 1983, reviewed existing evidence and scientific opinion. The federal panel concluded that obesity "is a killing disease that should receive the same medical attention" as other leading causes of death, and that thus far, "insufficient research attention had been paid to obesity as a risk to mental and physical health." Beyond the undeniable fact of risk, though, the panel found no substantial conclusions as to what actually causes overweight. Treatment was not even discussed.[3]

The Health Risks of Overweight ————————————

It is abundantly clear that overweight is one of America's—and the world's—leading health problems. In any given week, the *New York Times Sunday Book Review*'s list of the top ten non-fiction bestsellers will include at least two or three books on how to lose weight. Many of these books hit the top of the list and stay there for weeks.

Despite all the literature and all the studies, Americans in the 1980s are fatter than ever before. Nationally, we weigh more in all age groups than twenty years ago, with a gain of over 10 pounds in some age groups.[4] Depending upon whose figures one chooses, there are anywhere from 34 million to 80 million seriously overweight adults in the United States. Common estimates indicate that up to 50 percent of American adults and 10 percent to 20 percent of the children are overweight. The National Center for Health Statistics says that the average adult American male is now 20 to 30 pounds overweight.

At any one time, 40 million Americans are on some type of weight-loss diet. True *obesity*, which is defined as being more than 20 percent heavier than one's "ideal weight" (a figure which is itself not without controversy),[5] is said to afflict 20 million to 40 million Americans, with over 11 million considered to be severely obese.

Aside from the obvious physical and emotional discomforts, being overweight poses serious risks to health. As a frequently cited example, a 50-year-old man who is 50 pounds overweight has a 50 percent reduction in his life expectancy. The two most common risks associated with overweight are the greatly increased tendencies for Type II diabetes, and for elevated blood pressure and serum cholesterol levels. It is still not known exactly what links these conditions to overweight—which problem causes which, for example, or how—but in the majority of cases a reduction of weight will be automatically accompanied with a reduction of the associated problems.

Other increased health risks to the overweight include a greater likelihood of gallbladder stones, hernia, menstrual irregularity, problems with pregnancy (such as toxemia or gestational diabetes), a greater tendency for skin infections and varicose veins, liver disease, and some types of cancer—particularly, common cancers such as cancer of the prostate, breast, uterus, colon, or rectum. In addition, overweight can cause respiratory difficulties, leading to the retention of excessive carbon dioxide. The resulting sleepiness and lack of mental alertness is probably the leading reason why overly fat people are often thought of as mentally sluggish.[6] Finally, the burden of excessive weight makes obese people far more prone to disabling osteoarthritis, particularly of the knees, hips, and lower spine.

The problem of overweight, in fact, is such a critical issue that the U.S. Senate's landmark 1977 report *Dietary Goals for the United States* made "To Avoid Overweight" its first of seven major national goals. In that report, Dr. Beverly Winikoff, of the Rockefeller Foundation, stated that "obesity is probably the most common and one of the most serious nutritional problems affecting Americans today."[7] In the same report, Dr. Winikoff also noted the "staggering implications" of current research on preventing overweight through dietary change: even a 20 percent reduction in incidence would result in a minimum of 140,000 American lives saved annually. Hippocrates' famous dictum holds as true today as it did in ancient Greece, and for immeasurably greater numbers of people: "the fat die sooner than the thin."

The Outlook on Treatment

Not surprisingly, weight loss—or at least the promise of weight loss—has become big business. The "Fat Industry" has been estimated at $10 billion per year (over $200 million of this in over-the-counter drugs), not including the sales of popular diet books. At least a million people per year sign up for Weight Watchers or similar diet programs. Many of the most popular diet programs are notoriously ineffective (an estimated two percent of enrollees are still slim after seven years), and some can actually be quite dangerous. This includes diets that advocate a high protein, high fat, and low carbohydrate intake, including the infamous "liquid protein" diet.

Most attempts to reduce through a popular weight-loss program result in an all-too-familiar pattern: vigorous attempts to exercise and diet are rewarded by a short-term loss of weight, only to see the excess weight return soon after finishing the program. This commonplace experience led one physician to describe popular weight-loss programs as "the rhythm method of girth control."[8]

More dramatic measures are sometimes employed in cases of extreme obesity. These include *gastric restriction*—stapling closed a portion of the stomach so it can hold only a small volume of food (or in a newer version, inflating a balloon in the stomach to crowd its interior)—and *jejunoileal bypass*, a surgical process pioneered some thirty years ago, in which a portion of the small intestine is bypassed, resulting in weight loss due to malabsorption. Both operations commonly yield complications, and are avoided when possible.

Another technique, *suction lipectomy*, has grown more popular recently. This is a purely cosmetic process (and at $2,500 to $5,000 per operation, a luxuriously expensive one), in which excess fat is literally sucked out from under the skin by a vacuum tube.

Beyond these fairly brutal methods, a wide range of sophisticated pharmaceutical techniques are now being hotly pursued in hopes of winning big in the "Fat Industry." These approaches are working with substances such as *sucrose polyester*, an artificial fat used in cooking; artificial adrenaline, artificial insulin, and other artificial hormones, aimed at altering the metabolism in favor of fat loss; artificial drugs to interfere with the internal awareness of hunger; and the infamous *starch blockers*, which are designed to act by preventing the normal absorption of carbohydrates. According to a 1984 study in the *American Journal of Clinical Nutrition*, "More than 200 different starch blocker products have flooded the market over the past two years and were consumed at the rate of 1 million tablets per day."[9] However, the study also found that not only were these products ineffective in achieving their aims, but that they may contribute to damage to the intestinal lining, and even lead in the long run to greater weight gain rather than less.

Anorexia Nervosa and Bulimia

The problem of weight control has intensified in the past decade with the sudden escalation of two extreme eating disorders, largely among college-age women. *Anorexia nervosa*, a syndrome of pathological discipline and self-starvation, is not a new disorder. But just as the deaths of national figures such as Hubert Humphrey, John Wayne, and Rock Hudson have changed the national consciousness about cancer and AIDS, the tragic death of the young popular singer Karen Carpenter brought anorexia nervosa into sharper public view. Though not quite as well known, the related syndromes known collectively as *bulimia*, most commonly a pattern of overeating meals of staggering proportions followed by prolonged self-induced vomiting to avoid the attendant weight gain, have also begun to gain national attention.

As with obesity, estimates of the incidence of anorexia nervosa and bulimia vary. One study of college-age women found that between one-quarter and one-third of these women were involved in some level of these widespread eating disorders. One researcher puts the mortality rate of anorexia at a shocking 15 percent, explaining that the usual methods of psychotherapy generally do not seem to work.

While statistically of tiny incidence when compared with obesity, these two disorders have sent ripples of shock through the public and professional worlds alike. Unlike obesity, which is often perceived simply as being ungainly, the seemingly irrational character of anorexia and bulimia presents a frightening picture to the general populace, and even to those whose professional charge it is to treat these patients. (One specialist in eating disorders related sending out over two thousand invitations to capable therapists for a conference in approaches to treatment. He received only seven replies.[10])

The spectacle of anorexia and bulimia strike deep to our core, perhaps because they vividly illustrate the terrifying possibility of a humanity deeply out of control. Through the process called *psychic numbing*, it is easy for many to disassociate themselves from the news of starving masses in distant lands. And the fact that our own nation carries as much as seven or eight billion extra pounds of body fat can be dismissed from our minds as an abstraction. But one cannot easily forget the image of a highly intelligent, articulate, apparently happy college coed, stubbornly starving herself to death for no obvious reason. Anorexia and bulimia show us that in a sense, we as a civilization have lost control of ourselves, our patterns of consumption, and our ability to take rational steps to ensure our very survival.

With anorexia nervosa and bulimia at its extreme ends, and obesity, with all its associated potentially lethal risks, lying at the center, the broad spectrum of human problems classified as *eating disorders* represents a crisis in human civilization, a crisis of profound implications and epic dimensions. Despite advancements in theoretical research and more extreme forms of "treatment," there has been no slowing of these alarming trends.

Even so, within the confusion of conflicting scientific views and battling popular methods, some bright lights have begun to emerge. We will review this in Chapter 4 in the section titled "The Emerging Commonsense Perspective." The recent progress made in some quarters has yet to have much impact on America's weight problems. But positive strides are being taken to sort through the mass of research and clinical experiences, and to arrive at some simple conclusions. The problem with these encouraging developments is that they do not go far enough. They do not address the central issues of this epidemic, nor provide an appropriately thorough prescription for modern society.

The practical gains made by some therapists and practitioners have too often been one-sided, limited by the viewpoint that their particular approach contains "the key" to weight control, whether it be diet, exercise, or behavior modification. Others have put forth suggestions that are too vague and generalized to be of far-reaching value. Scientific research has tended to focus on the minute details, the *microscopic* aspects of what takes place in the human body and psyche. What has been lacking is a *macroscopic* view, a comprehensive, unifying understanding of life and human experience. Such a comprehensive perspective is the purpose of macrobiotics.

The Macrobiotic Approach to Life ——————————

Though popularly known simply as a diet, macrobiotics is better
described as a dietary philosophy. It is an embracing approach to living
with roots deep in traditional cultures of both the East and the West.
From the Greek *makro* (large) and *bios* (life), the term literally means
"longevity" and has also been translated as "living according to a large
view of life." Macrobiotics is not a specific "diet" in the modern sense;
it is a way of living based upon a natural dietary ecology. This means
that macrobiotics approaches the question of what we should eat, not
only in terms of how specific foods affect our bodies, but also in terms
of how our diet links us to the environment around us.

People often ask, "What is the difference between macrobiotics and
Further, an individual human being represents a complex ecology as
well. In addition to our mechanical and physiological functions, our
mental, emotional, intellectual, and spiritual faculties all play a part in
our own body ecology. All these levels of our existence play a part in
our health, and all interact with our daily eating and drinking. The
dietary principles of macrobiotics are described in detail in later chapters.

People often ask, "What is the difference between macrobiotics and
nutrition? Aren't they the same thing?" *Nutrition*, the study of food's
individual, separate physical components (fats, vitamins, amino acids,
and so forth) is an exciting and valuable field of science, but it represents
only a fragmentary part of the true study of food. In this sense, nutrition
might be termed *micro*biotics. Knowledge of the physical mechanics of
a vibrating violin string cannot explain the majesty of a great symphony;
likewise, nutritional science alone cannot realistically hope to unravel the
dietary and health behavior of a nation.

The Meaning of Food ——————————————

Beginning from a macrobiotic perspective, we must first realize that life
does not exist in a vacuum. We are in constant exchange with our
environment. In the process of living, we absorb nourishment from the
environment on many levels, including solid food, liquid, and gasses, and
the more subtle but equally crucial nourishment of light, heat, and the
full range of vibrations and waves filling the space around us. As we use
these absorbed features of our surroundings to animate our lives, we also
return unneeded and processed nourishment back to the environment,
in the form of solid, liquid, and, gaseous "waste," the caloric heat emana-
tions of activity, and the various vibrations and waves of our behavior,
expression, and thinking.

From this larger perspective, it is clear that the world of nature is as essential to human life as our own digestive systems, hearts, muscles, and brains. If deprived of any of these natural functions, whether of our "inner" physiological selves or our "outer" environmental selves, we would cease to exist.

Obviously, our lives depend on food; one might also say that a car could not run without being given gas—but the analogy is not complete. For our food is far more than mere *fuel*. Food is the means by which we carve out portions of the environment and make them into our own selves.

A painter surveys the landscape, selects appropriate portions of it, prepares an image of it, and serves it on a canvas for us to absorb through our sense of sight. But a good cook is a far more magical artist. A cook likewise surveys the landscape and chooses the appropriate portions for his or her "subject." Then the cook prepares those portions of the landscape themselves, and not merely a visual image, on the canvas of the kitchen stove. When we are served, we completely digest the "painting," and it actually forms the cells of which our blood, body, and brain are made. Let's see how this process takes place.

How Our Food Creates Us

In the course of eating, we are taking apart our food in various ways. This dissolving process actually starts with cooking, which begins to soften hard tissues and makes foods more digestible. It continues through the mechanical action of chewing and the electrochemical action of starch-digesting enzymes, called *amylases*, in saliva. When food reaches the stomach it is further dissolved by strong stomach acids and protein-digesting enzymes, notably *pepsin*. As food enters the *duodenum*, the connecting area between the stomach and small intestine, it is bathed in bile from the liver and gallbladder, and in pancreatic digestive fluids. *Bile* acts on fats, emulsifying them (dissolving them into smaller particles) so they can be more easily digested; and *pancreatic enzymes* act on proteins and carbohydrates as well as on fats.

At this point, a physiologist would consider our food as still being on the "outside" of ourselves. Though it is deep within our body, it still is no more absorbed into our own personal chemistry than if it were sitting in our hand or touching our skin. (There are exceptions; some strong substances such as alcohol, simple sugars, or spices are often absorbed through the lining of the mouth or stomach before this point.) It is only after food enters the intestinal tract that it takes the next step towards becoming part of us.

In the small intestine, many of the now-digested food particles come into contact with the intestinal *villi*, which are tiny, porous protuberances that allow minute food particles to pass through the intestine's wall and enter the blood supply. This entry is prepared and assisted by the millions of microorganisms—bacteria, yeasts, and other primitive life forms—that dwell in the intestine for just this purpose. These *intestinal flora* are in many ways similar to the microorganisms involved in infections, but while infectious germs are involved in the process of breaking down excessive nutrients that are attempting to get *out* of the body,[11] the intestinal microorganisms are breaking down nutrients to assist in their entry *into* the body.

Once "inside," the absorbed nourishment travels through our bloodstream. The newly enriched blood is carried first to the liver, where it is evaluated and chemically altered in dozens of ways to fine-tune its exact composition to suit the body's needs at that time. For example, unneeded sugars may be moved into storage or rerouted to become *triglycerides*, a special combination of fats found in humans and animals. Free amino acids may be synthesized into new complete proteins to help rebuild a structure elsewhere in the body. The fine-tuned blood is then carried to the heart and lungs to gather oxygen and physical pressure for circulation throughout the body. During the course of its circulation, the blood is continually routed through special filtering circuits that allow the kidneys and the pancreas and other endocrine glands to constantly adjust its composition, so it always suits our needs most precisely.

Finally, blood is passed through ever finer vessels (*capillaries*) until it comes into contact with individual body cells. At the cellular level, the nourishment of our food reaches its ultimate destination. On entering a cell, some of the nutrients' stored energies are released and used for our own activity. Some of the substance of the cell is used to create new tissue and repair or remold old, dying, and destroyed tissue. It is here that food finally "becomes us"—our substance, our energy, and our activity. Unlike the King's horses and King's men of the famous nursery rhyme, our bodies *do* "put it all back together again." Our food is reduced from its original structure as plants, animals, and other features of the environment, dissolved into its microscopic essence, and miraculously reassembled into an entirely new form—ourselves.

It is not only calories and structural proteins that are provided. There are also less obviously measurable *qualities* of our foods that transfer into our cells. And these more subtle qualitative differences between different foods profoundly affect our metabolism, behavior, and even our thinking. For example, we may receive 500 calories by consuming a certain portion of either carrots, table sugar, or alcohol. According to physical *quantitative* measurement, these three provide equivalent energy.

But we will experience these 500 calories very differently.

Because of their different natures, each of these foods will metabolize in dramatically different ways, and therefore produce very different behavioral tendencies. Or, as another example, we can obtain the recommended daily allotment of protein exclusively from either animal or vegetable sources. Again, the physical protein gram count may be identical, but as most vegetarians are aware, they produce a very different experience.

In a very literal sense, we are what we eat. Or more precisely, we are accurate reflections of the environment in which we live, as transferred from our "outer selves" to our "inner selves" through the process of food.

The Spiral of Creation

If we come from our food, then from where does our food originate? All animate life derives its existence from the elements of nature—the soil, water, sky, and minerals of the earth, and beyond these molecular worlds, from the energies of the sun. We ourselves are not equipped to absorb these natural "nutrients" directly, but the plant world can, and does. Through the processes of *photosynthesis* and *biosynthesis*, plants build themselves directly from the elements of nature and sunlight, and we assemble and maintain ourselves on those sources indirectly through plants. (Even carnivorous animals rely indirectly on the plant world, as it is ultimately plants that nourish the animal life which they eat.)

It is the same with a nursing infant. An infant cannot eat his environmental foods directly, but his mother can. Indirectly, the infant absorbs his environment through the medium of his mother. Likewise, we create ourselves and our lives out of the world of nature, though indirectly, by "nursing" on the plant world.

The elements of nature and the energies of the sun, in turn, are created and maintained by a larger, unseen world of *free energy*—high speed radiation and waves that emanate from the furthest reaches of the universe. The existence of energy itself is generated by the dynamics of *universal polarity*, the tendency of opposing and mutually attracting characters that underlies all phenomena. This polarizing tendency has been referred to throughout human history by many terms, such as Heaven and Earth, alpha and omega, dark and light, or yin and yang. (We will take a detailed look at the idea of yin and yang in Chapter 2.) Finally, the tendencies of polarity themselves are constantly arising out of the infinite expanse of the universe itself. This universal source is difficult for many of us to imagine, but we intuitively know of its existence. It has been described by such absolute terms as the One, the All-In-All, the Tao, and God.

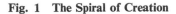

Fig. 1 The Spiral of Creation

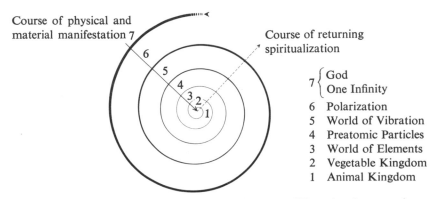

Course of physical and material manifestation 7

Course of returning spiritualization

7 {God / One Infinity
6 Polarization
5 World of Vibration
4 Preatomic Particles
3 World of Elements
2 Vegetable Kingdom
1 Animal Kingdom

The space outside of the spiral is the unmanifested, undifferentiated ocean of Infinity, and the worlds within the spiral are the relative and ephemeral worlds.

These various stages or levels of life can be pictured as one huge spiral of development, which we describe as the *Spiral of Creation*. Within this vast spirallic process, each realm of life arises as a condensation and more intensely organized transformation of the next larger realm that embraces and constantly nourishes it. Though we can divide the spectrum of life in this way, this division is not an absolute one. Each realm is distinct from the others, yet they are all intimately connected in one, great, continuous process of creation. According to this macroscopic view, it becomes clear that food is more than merely our fuel, just as an infant's mother represents far more in his life than a source of calories and protein.

The Separation of Modern Humanity ━━━━━━━

Human civilization has developed and flourished within the context of this vast, ongoing spirallic process, with food always serving as the source point linking us to the environment that produced us. Historically, the issue of food supply has always served as the economic pivot on which a society's destiny turns. As the prime economic determinant, food has dictated great migrations and changed trade patterns, and has formed the underpinnings of our daily way of life. Just as individual human lives are directed by the governing force of food, so has the social fabric been woven of threads spun by our environment, through our everyday food and drink. In the drama of human life, we are but the actors, while God and the universe are the playwrights—food and the environment are the directors.

In the present era, this intimate connection has been broken. With the advent of industrialization, we have suddenly fashioned entirely new patterns of culture, economy, agriculture, diet, and lifestyle. The formation of centralized urban and suburban living has removed over 98 percent of us from direct contact with the land. We have insulated ourselves from our food's real nature with extensive processing and artificial production techniques.

At nearly any time in history, an average meal would represent the unadulterated yield of our local environment, assisted by our own labors or the work of perhaps a handful of others. An average meal today is likely to contain the labors of thousands of people throughout the continent, and sometimes from even further away, in its growing, processing, packaging, transport, financing, marketing, and preparation.

In *The Next Economy*, social economist Paul Hawken describes this situation: "From an agrarian society, where economic production was largely self-sufficient and where people spent most of their time producing necessities for themselves, we have become a people who perform only tiny segments of the overall task of production, and we consume mostly what has been produced by others."[12] ". . . The process of growing the food we eat . . . [now] requires the skills of many different persons, from graphic designers of packages to room-service maids, from roustabouts to waitresses, from chemical engineers to metallurgists."[13] As Hawken points out, it cost from $3,000 to $5,000 in 1982 to ship a truckload of lettuce from California to the East Coast, and at considerable expense to the environment along the way.

And what quality of food does this process produce? Even without taking into account the details of how our nutritional pattern has been drastically altered, which we will look at in the next chapter, it is all too obvious that our diet is something unique in history. This is well expressed in the 1978 report *The Changing American Diet*: "If our great-grandparents spent a day eating with us, they would be wide-eyed and shocked. And if they were plopped down in a modern supermarket, they would probably not know for sure whether they were in a toy store, hardware store or grocery store."[14] Considering what we are eating, it is no wonder we tend to feel confused or fragmented in today's world!

The Source of Eating Disorders ───────────

People are often surprised to learn that obesity is quite rare in traditional and agricultural societies. Perhaps we have unquestioningly accepted popular images of the plump farmer, or the fat African chieftain. But these images have little basis in historical reality. In fact, modern research has revealed that obesity always appears rather suddenly and establishes itself as a common condition *simultaneously* with the appearance of affluence and modern eating habits.[15] This is certainly no coincidence. Nor is it a coincidence that the first documented case of anorexia nervosa happened in the same place (England) and at almost precisely the same time (the late 1600s) as the emergence of obesity as a common occurrence *and* the first historical documentation in the Western world of diabetes.[16] It should come as no suprise that bulimia is also a disorder that appears almost exclusively in modernized, affluent societies.

Overweight and eating disorders cannot be explained solely by examining our internal physiological structures, or our personal psyches and family backgrounds. They represent a more pervasive problem with the way we as a society interact with our natural surroundings. As we isolate ourselves from nature and natural patterns, our sense of who we are loses its natural clarity. In the modern world, this gap has widened into a vast chasm.

Socially, this disorientation manifests in such expressions as an agriculture that depletes its soil and weakens its crops in the name of progress; as a technology that devastates its natural resources and displaces millions of native residents in the name of productivity; and as a military policy that prepares for the destruction of the planet's entire ecosystem in the name of defense. Individually, we recognize these behaviors as chaotic—we might even say, as dangerously insane. But we are unable to discover how to change our course, because we don't realize where our original roots to a more sound, truly productive way of living were severed.

On an individual level, this widening gap between humanity and nature has resulted, not only in the common feeling of alienation, but also in the weakening of our natural sense of food. Overweight, obesity, anorexia nervosa, and bulimia are symptoms of this loss. Recovery from these problems is possible, and it needs to begin with our recovering our sense of the natural order of diet.

[1] "Dieting: The Losing Game," *Time*, January 20, 1986, p. 55.

[2] *Eating Disorders*, Hilde Bruch, MD, p. 17.

[3] "Federal Panel Issues Warning of Obesity Peril," *The Oregonian*, February 14, 1985; and "Society Abhors Obesity," *The Hartford Courant*, February 23, 1985.

[4] "The Roots of Gluttony," Konner, Melvin, *Science Digest*, September 1982.

[5] See discussion at the beginning of Chapter 5.

[6] *Human Nutrition and Dietetics*, London, 1979, pp. 241 ff.

[7] *Dietary Goals for the United States*, Select Committee on Nutrition and Human Needs, p. 7.

[8] *Dietary Goals*, p. 9.

[9] The American Journal of Clinical Nutrition, February 1984, pp. 196–200.

[10] Dr. Steven Levenkron, *Treating and Overcoming Anorexia Nervosa*, p. xi.

[11] See "The Progressive Development of Illness" in Chapter 5.

[12] *The Next Economy*, Paul Hawken, p. 117.

[13] Hawken, p. 20.

[14] *The Changing American Diet*, Center for Science in the Public Interest, 1978.

[15] *The Emergence of Western Diseases*, H. Trowell and D. Burkitt, p. 14 ff.

[16] *Diabetes and Hypoglycemia*, p. 46 ff.

2. The Natural Order of Diet ▬▬▬▬

There is scarcely any word that triggers more connotations, both positive and negative, to the modern mind than the word "diet." Possibly the most common feeling is that this is a four-letter word that implies deprivation, the loss of favorite pleasures, and will power of impossible dimensions. Many modern quick-weight-loss diets have earned such poor reputations (and often deservedly so), that an article in the journal *Medical Self-Care* addressed the question of how to lose weight with a two-word headline: Stop Dieting.

As our understanding of nature and food has declined, so has the definition of the word "diet" grown increasingly narrow. While today it is mostly confined to mean a restricted regimen of specific foods in specific volumes, with specifically prohibited foods, it was originally quite a different concept. The Greek word *diaita*, from which our "diet" is derived, was apparently coined by Hippocrates, the founder of Western medicine. Hippocrates' form of medicine was broad-based and wholistic, and relied on naturally prepared simple foods as the treatment of choice. Hippocrates used the term *diaita* to refer to a *way of living life* harmoniously, with particular care to the selection and preparation of the proper foods.

This is what is meant when we refer to the macrobiotic approach to diet. Proper diet consists of more than consuming the best quality of ingredients. It also means putting one's life in order, and learning to choose, balance, prepare and consume the most appropriate foods for creating that life.

Since persons who suffer from eating disorders often experience obsessive thoughts, fears, or other fragmented and unbalanced attitudes toward food, it is important that we achieve the broadest understanding of diet as a foundation for recovery. This chapter considers seven general aspects of the natural order of diet.

1. The Evolutionary and Physiological Order of Diet –

As we saw in the previous chapter, the vegetable and animal kingdoms represent the last two stages of life's condensing spiral of development. Within the animal world, some species create themselves *directly* by consuming plants exclusively (*herbivores*), while others secure their plant foods *indirectly* by consuming other animals (*carnivores*). Still others have the capacity to create themselves through both means; we ourselves belong to this *omnivorous* category.

However, while we are physiologically *able* to derive nourishment from animal foods, we usually compromise our health in doing so. This is because, from the standpoint of physiology, we are much closer to the design of true herbivores than true carnivores.

Our saliva, for example, contains amylases, which are enzymes that assist the digestion of complex carbohydrate (also referred to as *starch*). Since carbohydrates are available almost exclusively from vegetable sources, a carnivore has no use for amylase. This is the reason animals like cows, deer, and giraffe chew their food at length, while dogs, cats, and wolves simply tear and swallow. (The way in which individual humans eat often suggests which dietary pattern they have adopted!)

The structure of the human digestive system also reflects more of a herbivorous than carnivorous balance. We have lengthy intestinal tracts, which allow food to remain for longer than twenty-four hours before elimination. This is normal for an herbivore, but would be dangerous for a carnivore. Animal foods putrefy far more quickly than vegetable foods, producing potentially toxic substances as they decay. Because of this, a true carnivore's digestive tract is designed to hold food for a long time in the stomach, where it is bathed in strong acids, and to pass through a short intestinal tract in a much briefer time.

Even our teeth reflect our essentially plant-eating design. Among an adult's thirty-two teeth, only four are "biting and tearing" teeth (*canines*), while our eight front teeth are adapted to slicing or chopping, and our twenty back teeth, the majority, are "grinders" best suited to crushing foods such as nuts, seeds, grains, and tougher roots. Taking this proportion as a model would suggest that our diet might safely include up to one-eighth animal foods, one-quarter plant foods that are easily chopped (such as leafy vegetables and fruits), and over one-half grains, seeds, nuts, and hardier, tougher plant foods. Further, since the continuous grinding of a food mixes it more thoroughly with saliva, it would seem we are designed to include complex carbohydrate foods as more than half of our diet.

This physiological preference for carbohydrate-rich plant foods is also reflected in our development as a species. Each species of animal shows a preference for the foods that most represent the environment that existed during the epoch of that animal's own development. For example, the various species of giant reptiles co-existed with the gigantic, lush foliage of their era, while the smaller, more dense forms of modern vegetable plants, nuts, seeds, and fruits gave rise, respectively, to families of mammals, squirrels, birds, and apes. The most recent botanical arrivals, and nutritionally the most complex, have been the cereal grains and modern seed plants. It was during this epoch that the human form finally emerged, and accordingly, cereals have been the staple food of human civilization throughout our history.

Fig. 2   Proportion of Human Teeth

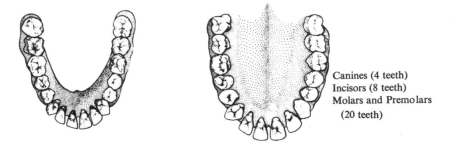

Canines (4 teeth)
Incisors (8 teeth)
Molars and Premolars
(20 teeth)

Thus, while we are physically capable of eating almost anything under the sun without immediate repercussions, we are most suited to a diet that is mostly or completely vegetarian, high in complex-carbohydrate foods, and particularly revolving around cereal grains.

2.   The Metabolic Order of Diet

In studying the effects of different diets on human metabolism, we need to consider three factors. First, what nutrients we require, and in what proportion. Second, what food sources contain these nutrients, especially in as close to ideal proportions as possible. And finally, how efficiently we are able to use the nutrients of different foods, including the question of how much toxic waste they produce when metabolized.

The three classes of nutrients which we require in the largest amounts are called *macronutrients*; in descending order of amount needed, these are carbohydrate, protein, and fat. (The term *micronutrients* refers to minerals, vitamins, enzymes, and other components of diet which we need in tiny amounts.)

Carbohydrate: The prime function of carbohydrate is energy; carbohydrate is our preferred source of calories. As it is digested, carbohydrate is reduced to a simplified form called *glucose*, which is used directly by our bodies' cells as fuel. Both protein and fat can also supply energy, so why is carbohydrate preferred? Simply speaking, carbohydrate (particularly complex carbohydrate) "burns the cleanest," that is, it produces very little toxic waste.

There are essentially three types of carbohydrate: *complex carbohydrates* (also called *starches* or *polysaccharides*), which are found in whole grains, beans, nuts and seeds, and most vegetables; *simple carbohydrates* (also called *sugars*, *simple sugars*, and *mono-* or *di-saccharides*), which naturally occur in fruits, honey, maple sap and other naturally sweet foods; and *refined carbohydrates*, which include processed foods such as table sugar, commercial corn syrup and fructose, white flour and white rice, and other refined grain products.

Of these, complex carbohydrates are the highest quality energy source. One reason is that the long process of breaking the complex starch chains down to glucose gives the body a chance to continually balance its metabolic reactions. Simple sugars and refined starches break down more rapidly or in an uneven manner, often producing extreme swings in our internal reactions.[1] Another reason is that the foods that contain complex carbohydrate often also contain a range of other nutrients, including protein and fats (oils), and minerals and vitamins which help us metabolize the starch itself.

This is an important reason why fruits, though they are a "natural food," are not an ideal food as a prime energy source. They usually require additional sources of minerals and some vitamins (especially B vitamins) to balance their effects in the body. (What often happens with excessive fruit consumption, in fact, is that a large part of the sugars in fruits is converted by the body to triglycerides, rather than used as energy.) The same is obviously the case with refined carbohydrates, and even with those that have been "enriched." There is increasing evidence that the body cannot accept and utilize the vitamins and minerals that are artificially reintroduced into "enriched" foods, as it can those which naturally occur in the unrefined products.

Protein: The primary function of protein in our diet is as a structural substance rather than energy source. Our bodies are composed primarily of protein (that is, the solid portion of our bodies, discounting the large amount of water of which we are made). Dietary protein is ideally used to build new muscle or organ tissue, or to replace worn out tissues. A minute but crucially important amount of dietary protein goes into building new enzymes and hormones.

When we are starved of carbohydrate, we can draw on our protein supply for calories. However, there are two problems with this. Before proteins can be changed to glucose they must be *deaminated*, that is, their component amino acids are stripped away, broken down, and changed into fat. The nitrogen that is left from this process is converted into ammonia, which is further converted into *urea*, the chief end-product of the decomposition of proteins. Urea is diluted in our urine. Since these protein by-products are highly acidic, they represent toxic wastes that consume a lot of energy and use extra minerals to neutralize and excrete. They can cause damage if they build up to excessive levels. This is one reason why "high-protein" diets are potentially dangerous.

The second problem with using protein for energy is that this draws on our supply of amino acids, making them unavailable for their normal body-building purposes. This is the reason for the wasting of muscle and organ deterioration seen in victims of prolonged starvation. The only way to avoid this is to consume a large proportion of protein, which returns us to the problem described in the last paragraph. Obviously, protein can be safely used for energy only in small amounts and for short periods.

Protein from plant sources is considered nutritionally superior to protein from animal sources, because it generally is *not* accompanied by the saturated fats that are found in animal foods. This brings us to the next macronutrient.

Fat: Fat's primary purpose is as a specialized form of energy. Fat is the primary means animals use to store reserves of energy. However, fat produces highly toxic, acid wastes when it is metabolized; this is especially true when fat is "burned" in the absence of glucose. Therefore, while fat is the most efficient form of energy *storage* for reserves, it is not necessarily the most ideal form of ongoing energy supply. In fact, warnings concerning the dangers of fat intake have become one of the few points on which nearly all health experts agree.

The degree to which a fat is *saturated* refers to the fact that a fat molecule has many potential chemical bonding points on its surface. In a *polyunsaturated* fat, such as the oils found in vegetables and grains, these bonding sites are open, which gives the molecule more metabolic flexibility. In a *saturated* fat these sites are occupied by hydrogen atoms, making the molecule less subject to changes in the body. (Artifically *hydrogenated* oils, though they are of vegetable origin, behave much the same as naturally occurring saturated fats.) An excess of *any* type of dietary fat has proven to be dangerous, but our bodies can more easily make constructive use of polyunsaturated fats than saturated fats.

An important point to realize is that, while a certain amount of fat is necessary in the body, it needn't be consumed directly as dietary fat. Both carbohydrate and protein are regularly converted by the liver into body fat. Theoretically, we could exist and enjoy excellent health with practically no fat in our diet. However this is unlikely to happen. Any diet containing animal foods, even so-called "lean" or "low-fat" animal or dairy products, will of course be fairly rich in fats. But further, any plant-based diet that includes grains or even small amounts of beans, nuts, or seeds will furnish plenty of fats in the form of vegetable oils.

The Ideal Balance of Nutrients

Until the last decade, much of the twentieth century's nutritional viewpoint was based on pioneering research centering in Germany in the nineteenth century. This early nutritional work emphasized the importance of protein, and particularly animal protein. This viewpoint most likely arose from the fact that the "normal" diet at that time and in that locale was high in animal foods. Thus, even though a significant majority of human civilization throughout history has subsisted on diets containing little or no animal products, and there is no scientific or practical reason why we should not also do so (quite the contrary, in fact), we still see "meats" and "dairy products" often referred to as two of "the four basic food groups." In historical terms, as we shall see in the next section, this is patent nonsense; nor is it defensible in metabolic terms.

It has been only in the past ten years that we seem to be successfully getting away from this blatantly cultural bias, and readjusting our dietary priorities to more accurately fit the facts. The pioneering work of the U.S. Senate's *Dietary Goals* in 1977 recommended that we strive as a nation to adopt the following guidelines, measured as percentages of our total daily calorie intake:

1. Complex carbohydrates and other natural sugars should be nearly doubled, increasing from 28 percent to 48 percent.
2. Refined and processed sugars should be reduced from 45 percent to about 10 percent.
3. Overall fat intake should be cut from 40 percent to 30 percent, with saturated and mono-unsaturated fats reduced from 35 percent to 20 percent, and polyunsaturated fats increased from 7 percent to 10 percent.
   There was no change in protein percentages recommended; the average American diet was found to contain about 12 percent protein.

The report then translated these goals into dietary terms: *reduce* the use of refined foods, fat, and many animal products, and *increase* the use of unrefined whole grains, fresh vegetables and fruits, and low fat animal products such as fish and poultry.

Since *Dietary Goals* first appeared, dozens of similar sets of guidelines have emerged from a wide range of scientific and governmental institutions, both in the United States and abroad, all offering the same general view of the ideal nutrition pattern. Many authorities have advanced the view that the goals should go even further, reducing, for example, the saturated fats portion to nearly zero and the overall fat intake to significantly less, reducing all animal foods further, and specifically increasing the proportion of grains and cereal foods. This viewpoint concurs with macrobiotic guidelines. Figure 3 shows the 1977 guidelines as compared with the then current pattern, and with a nutritional analysis of macrobiotic guidelines.

Fig. 3 Nutritional Comparision between the Current American Diet, the U.S. Dietary Goals, and the Standard Macrobiotic Diet

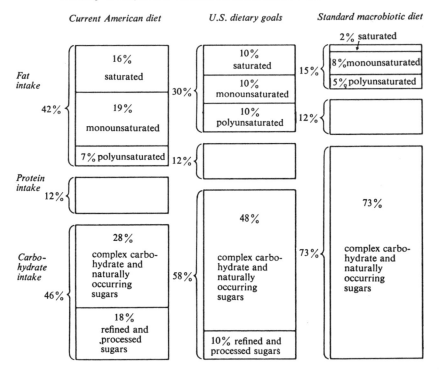

This pattern, as it turns out, is found to describe the diets of many ages-old dietary traditions, and this leads us to the next aspect of dietary order.

3. The Traditional and Historical Order of Diet ───────

Current research tells us that the nutritional pattern of macrobiotics was arrived at thousands of years ago, through many thousands of years of trial and error. Primitive hunter-gatherers, who preceded agricultural societies, obtained most of their food from plant sources.[2] Studies of contemporary hunting-gathering groups suggest that animal foods supplied 25 percent to 35 percent of their diet, with the remaining 65 percent to 75 percent furnished by the plant kingdom. In relation to the pattern we are recommending, these groups ate a diet somewhat higher in protein (15 percent to 20 percent rather than 12 percent), with 15 percent to 30 percent fat and 50 percent to 70 percent carbohydrate. This primitive diet included no added milk, sugar, salt, or alcohol, and of course, no refined or artificially processed foods.

With the "First Agricultural Revolution" some twelve thousand years ago, both agriculture and food storage methods were developed. The diet of the hunter-gatherers changed somewhat; the diet of the new "peasant-agriculturalists" *decreased* in protein to 10 percent to 15 percent, starch foods *increased* slightly to 60 percent to 75 percent, and fats probably *decreased* slightly to 10 percent to 15 percent. This pattern is strikingly similar to the macrobiotic nutritional guidelines outlined in Figure 3. Throughout history, problems frequently arose to interrupt this pattern, including droughts and famines, economic difficulties resulting in poor food supply or poor food production methods, and the uprooting and population shifts occasioned by wars and climatic changes. Nevertheless, this pattern remained the ideal for nearly twelve thousand years.

With the advent of the Industrial Revolution, this pattern began to change drastically. Newer methods of agriculture and food processing changed the nature of our basic foodstuffs. Increase in transportation and trade brought the widescale importation of non-local, previously "luxury" food items. Examples of this were coffee, tea, chocolate, sugar, and tropical fruits to northern Europe and the United States. Advances in refrigeration and ballooning affluence allowed a tremendous increase of animal and dairy food consumption. Improvements in mechanized milling and processing brought about the widespread refining of our staple foods, the cereal family, and the advent of commercialism thoroughly altered the family's traditional eating patterns with a new market of snack and convenience foods. By the 1950s, the common food pattern in the United States (and much of the rest of the world) had moved farther away from the traditional pattern than at any other time in history.

In the book *Diet and Nutrition: A Holistic Approach*, Dr. Rudolph Ballentine finds certain recurrent patterns of nutrition among widely different dietary traditions of what he terms the "stable" population groups throughout the world. In other words, in areas where people have been able to adapt to their environment and refine their way of living for many generations, we have always gravitated to a consistent way of eating.

He refers to this universal pattern as *Five Traditional Food Groups*, consisting of the following (in descending order by volume):

1. *Grains*, which "constitute the bulk of most of these diets and are consumed in the largest quantities";
2. *Vegetables*, generally fresh but cooked, and of course, selected from the locale and not imported;
3. *Beans and bean products* (such as tofu and tempeh), which supplement the protein and oils present in grains;
4. *The raw group*, which consists of small amounts of easily digested raw vegetables, presumably for the supplemental vitamins and enzymes they can provide, even when used only in small, garnish amounts;
5. What Ballantine calls the "B_{12} *group*," which may contain either very small amounts of supplemental animal food or some naturally fermented foods, such as natural pickles, miso, or tempeh.[3]

In addition to this basic pattern, Ballentine found that fruits "were often regarded as a luxury," and that animal foods came to play a prominent part only in areas where adverse climate or terrain made a more vegetarian diet impractical.[4] This pattern precisely describes what we are referring to as the standard macrobiotic dietary pattern.

4.   The Ecological and Economic Order of Diet ———

One of the most profound shifts produced by the changes described above has been an essentially economic one. Until the advent of the Industrial Revolution, certain foods were naturally seen as luxuries, while others were commonly available to all, as long as the crops were successful. This natural economic order is not man-made; it is a direct reflection of nature. Cereal grains and beans, for example, have historically been our most economical food crops. They lend themselves well to a sustainable agriculture and are easily stored. The land on which they are grown is used from eight to thirty times more efficiently when its products are used directly as food than when they are used as animal feed for a more carnivorous diet.[5]

Thus, meat, poultry, eggs, and especially dairy products have generally served as luxury items, while cereals and beans have been commoners' food. The only groups who have consistently been in a position to enjoy dietary luxuries on a regular basis have been the very wealthy (usually land-owners), royalty, and the high clergy. It is interesting to note that obesity has usually been limited to these three groups. (Perhaps it is not coincidental that the majority of the world's wars have been initiated by members of this dietary elite.)

Today the natural economic order is in chaos, so much so that foods' historical roles are often reversed. Those living in urban ghettos, for example, may live at the lowest average income levels while eating nothing but refined sugar, white flour, fatty meats, and milk—traditionally food only "for kings." And one may need to travel to a natural food store, located in a fairly affluent neighborhood, to find the humblest fare of organically, or non-technologically or "primitively" grown rice and beans!

Since the availability of foods has so drastically changed, it doesn't occur to most of us that such commonplace daily items as orange juice, tomatoes, spices, honey, and milk are tremendous luxuries. But they are. Even if they are currently cheap to buy, they are still "luxuries" in terms of the natural economy, to which our bodies have been adapted for tens of thousands of years. We need to look beyond the technologically altered economy existing today, and consider each food in terms of its place in nature's economy, because it is this order which our metabolisms respect. Though it may seem that we can "afford" to drink fresh cow's milk, eat steak, and have an orange every day, *physiologically*, we may be able to afford these special-occasion foods only once or twice per month, or per year.

The economic order also implies an *ecological* order. While *economical* means "what is readily available and most efficient to use," *ecological* suggests the idea of "what is most appropriate in this environment and maintains the health of the environment in the best way." Since energy-intensive, high-technology farming and factory processing harm the environment, their products are less ecological than simpler, small-scale organic agriculture and non-adulterated, whole foods.

"What is most appropriate" suggests that we eat foods that grow nearby, or that are adapted naturally to a similar climate. Ideally, we should select our foods from a 500 or 600 mile radius. Not only are these foods fresher and require less technology in their packing and shipping, they have also adapted themselves to our own climate as they have grown. Their precise mineral balance and moisture content, for example, may be very different than that of similar produce grown 2,000 miles away. Recall that we rely on the plant world to transform the sunshine, water, soil, and other elements of nature into substances we can consume. The ecological order simply means that plants in our own neighborhood will *feed* us our own neighborhood, and not one from a different environment.

Even at times when it is not possible or practical to eat foods that have literally grown nearby, we can at least select foods *in season*, and use primarily foods from a climate similar to our own. In Florida, for example, we can more easily use a slightly larger volume of warm-climate fruits than in Detroit (still remembering that on the whole, the role fruits play is more as a "luxury" than a staple).

Our cooking methods, too, reflect our climate and season, so that more well-cooked foods and less raw foods are generally used in the North and the winter, while the reverse may be true in the South and in the hot summer. Learning how to apply the principle of ecological order in our meals is one of the keys of mastering the art of macrobiotic cooking.

5.   The Behavioral and Psychological Order of Diet —

Our attitudes toward food and the role it plays in our lives have profoundly changed. In the past, we ate in order to live. In the modern world, we too often live in order to eat.

In *The Unsettling of America*, the noted farmer-philosopher Wendell Berry describes this change with rare insight. Berry points out that at the turn of the twentieth century the majority of the U.S. population was directly and personally involved in the production of food. This, of course, was as it had been throughout human history. At present, less than one century later, less than two percent of the population is involved with farming. This is the first time in history that the vast majority of people have been completely removed from the business of growing and harvesting our daily food. With this radical shift in human experience, we have ceased being a society of "producers," and have become the world's first few generations of "consumers," a role previously played only by select segments (and by far the minority) of any society. As Berry points out, this event has drastically changed the ways in which we view the land, ourselves, and each other. Above all, it has completely altered the everyday meaning of food.

Until this century, food had two basic "meanings." First, it represented our survival, our immediate means of living, and our partner in the game of life. Further, food represented our link with the soil and nature, our source and origin—in a fundamental way, our ecological "parents." In this connection, by the way, it is not surprising that eating disorders are frequently accompanied by disturbed or imbalanced parent-child relationships.

The first meaning is more economical, while the second might be called more psychological or more spiritual. And out of both economic common sense and this spiritual and ecological sense of our connection with nature, food was generally respected, at times even revered. Most traditional cultures represented cereal grains as a deity; the word "cereal," for example, derives from *Ceres*, the Romans' goddess of grain and the harvest. In some cultures the god or goddess of that culture's particular grain occupied the primary place of daily worship. In both Judaism and Christianity, prayer over the breaking of bread is still a central gesture of respect to the sanctity of the earth and nature's order.

A third meaning also existed for food: celebration. Food meant especially for fun and merry-making appeared during selected days of festivity. These were often the only times that nutritional luxuries were enjoyed. Such "special occasions" were, however, exactly that.

The modern consumer society, being effectively removed from the reality of the soil, has largely lost its direct sense of the first two meanings. Famine has not disappeared; quite the contrary. Large masses in the modern world do experience starvation. But the rest of society does not understand this experience in the way a land-based farming community does. In our cities, and even on American farms, our sense of immediate survival is tied not to the reality of crops but the reality of money. We do not starve from lack of food—it sits rotting in federally subsidized grain elevators—but from the unavailability of money. We as a civilization do not know where our food comes from. We have separated ourselves from our partner in life; we do not know who our "parents" are.

The third meaning, food as celebration, has meanwhile grown grossly out of proportion. We have come to know food as recreation, as entertainment. Food is advertised in the commercial media on the basis of its value as sensory gratification. Even for those who do not openly manifest one eating disorder or another, food has commonly taken on the nature of a drug. Books are beginning to appear on how to "Eat to Win" and how to choose foods that give the best advantage over an antagonist during a business lunch.

Paralleling the progressive distortion of our diet's nutritional, economic, and ecological profile, its "psychological profile" has grown equally chaotic. Figure 4 lists twenty-seven different "meanings of overeating" that have been reported by various researchers.[6]

36

Fig. 4   Twenty-Seven Different "Meanings" of Overeating

1. Diminishing anxiety
2. Achieving pleasure
3. Achieving social success and acceptance
4. Relieving frustration and deprivation
5. Expressing hostility (conscious or unconscious)
6. Diminishing feelings of insecurity
7. Self indulgence
8. Rewarding oneself
9. Expressing defiance
10. Submitting, e.g., to parental authority
11. Self punishment in response to guilt
12. Diminishing guilt
13. Exhibitionism
14. Attaining attention and care
15. Justifying failure in life
16. Testing love
17. Counteracting a feeling of being unloved
18. Distorting reality
19. Identifying with a fat person
20. Sedating oneself
21. Avoiding competition in life
22. Avoiding changing the status quo
23. Proving one's inferiority
24. Avoiding maturity [i.e., responsibility]
25. Diminishing fear of starvation
26. Consciously fulfilling the wish to be fat
27. Handling anxiety from infantile oral frustration

It goes without saying that most peasant-agriculturalists would find this list difficult to comprehend. Yet, this may be an accurate profile of the psychological trauma with which food is intertwined, for one-half or more of the modern population.

There are two other crucial aspects of the behavioral order of diet that have dramatically changed in this century. These are the human context of meals, and the balance between eating and activity. Concerning the context of meals, the Senate's *Dietary Goals* quoted noted child psychologist Bruno Bettelheim:

> Eating and being fed are intimately connected with our deepest feelings. They are the basic interactions between human beings on which rest all later evaluations of oneself, of the world, and of our relationship to it. Eating experiences condition our entire attitude to the world . . . Nothing is more divisive than when people eat a different fare, in different rooms.[7]

It is not only what foods we eat, but *how* we eat them, the eating experience itself, that affects us. When food is eaten calmly it is digested more completely than when eaten "on the run" or when one is upset, anxious, or angry. Our autonomic nervous system also tends to inhibit digestion when we are standing or walking, and orients the digestive organs toward efficient functioning only when we are sitting and relaxed.

In a natural context, meals are also a social exchange. The *Dietary Goals* go on to state, "At a time when more and more meals are being taken away from home, removed from the company of family members, perhaps [we should consider the possibility that this] substantially contributes to the stresses found in modern family life." In fact, we of this century have evolved entirely new habits of continuous snacking, eating on the run, and eating more fragmented diets as our patterns of family unity have begun to dissolve. And these new habits contribute not only to family "stresses," but to our own individual physiological and psychological wear and tear as well. It is worth nothing that persons who develop eating disorders often come to prefer solitude, even reclusion, during their mealtimes. In Chapter 8 we offer some guidelines, not on *what* to eat, but on *how* to eat.

Finally, the behavioral order of diet recognizes the importance of balancing our eating with our activity. Even if one consumes wonderfully healthy, macrobiotically prepared food, it will do little but turn to waste in the body if we do nothing!

During this century the actual volume of calories we consume has, on the average, not increased, but the amount of calories we actively use through physical activity has substantially *decreased*. There is also the question of the *quality* of our activity. For example, it is true that mental activity uses up a large amount of calories, which is why tremendous concentration can be physically exhausting. However, mental effort and physical effort place different nutritional demands upon us. The brain and nervous system burn calories exclusively from *glucose*, while the effort expended by moving our muscles will often use up calories from *fat*. A day of studying and a long walk may seem to have the same requirements on a "calorie chart," but their effects on our body and our diet are actually quite different.

Different types of physical activity place different demands on the body as well, according to such variables as the speed, pace, and rhythm of our movement. When choosing our meals, it is important to keep in mind just what kind of activity we will be doing. If we are more occupied with mental efforts our need for oils, protein, and fluids may be significantly less than for someone engaged in heavy physical labor. As a student of mine once remarked, it makes no sense for a young female office worker in an urban setting to eat the diet of a neolithic hunter.

It is not necessary to make an elaborate list of what kinds of activities are needed. The general principle is one of commonsense balance. Mental and physical activities need to balance each other. Some type of physical effort that uses the whole body in a harmonious way, such as walking, gardening, or house cleaning, helps to offset the unbalancing effects of a stressful, complicated lifestyle. This point brings us to the next aspect of natural dietary order.

6. The Individual and Intuitive Order of Diet ———————

One of the key principles of macrobiotic thought is that *everything is* unique. This certainly applies to people, and this is why it is so important to remember that dietary needs cannot be rigidly standardized. While there are general dietary principles that are common to all humanity, and others that apply to most people in a certain age bracket or specific climatic zone, everyone's specific dietary needs are unique. There is no one diet that is precisely right for everyone. Further, every individual's needs are constantly changing, and sometimes dramatically so.

A common difficulty we experience in writing or teaching about macrobiotics is that people often do not grasp this point. It is appropriate and necessary to present our dietary principles as actual guidelines, such as those found in this book or the menu suggestions given in the companion volume.[8] But these guidelines are only presented as average, generalized examples. In actual macrobiotic practice, our meals will naturally vary from person to person, day to day, and season to season.

For example, we need to consider our own particular dietary past. If we have recently (for the past months or even years) been consuming a large amount of salt, then our personal use of items such as *sea salt*, *natural soy sauce*, and *miso* (which contain some salt) should probably be carefully limited. After some years of eating macrobiotically, we will likely find that our need for these good quality mineral sources increases. Also, a past high intake of salt or of animal protein and fats may give us a greater need for fluid, as extra fluids are usually needed to help in their elimination. But it is impossible to say categorically that we need a certain number of glasses of water per day. After several months of eating a less salty, vegetarian diet, our natural requirement for fluid may substantially decrease. This is one reason it is often advisable to consult with an experienced macrobiotic teacher when adopting macrobiotic eating principles for health reasons.

The principle of universal uniqueness applies to foods, as well as to people. Not fully recognizing this fact is one of nutritional science's biggest mistakes: we cannot rigidly standardize foods or nutrients. Science attempts to express the behavior of foods by using scales of uniform measurement, such as calories, grams of protein, milligrams of vitamin C, or number of amino acids. But this approach is wholly inadequate; the relative failure of modern science to deal with problems such as obesity, diabetes, or anorexia nervosa stands as testimony.

For example, describing an individual's diet as containing a certain number of calories is a common practice in the effort to control weight. While this system has some limited usefulness for purposes of scientific discussion, it is virtually devoid of practical value in choosing an appropriate diet. This is self-evident; people who labor over calorie counting charts are not commonly successful in controlling their weight.

For one thing, one calorie each of table sugar, carrot, butter, and sesame oil will all behave very differently in our body. The same is true for an identical number of carbohydrate grams obtained from different food sources. As we explained in *Diabetes and Hypoglycemia*,[9] recent research has completely upset the conventional view that all complex carbohydrates have the same effect on the body. In fact, clinical trials in the past several years showed that dozens of different carbohydrate sources all elicited completely unique blood sugar responses. This discovery, which to our knowledge is still unexplained by modern science, invalidates much of the conventional nutritional treatment of diabetes and hypoglycemia.

The same can be said of the conventional viewpoint regarding calories and obesity. Scientific articles often make flat statements such as "[Overweight] occurs when food [that is, calorie] intake exceeds the energy [again, calorie] requirement of the body for physical activity and growth."[10] However, numerous surveys have found that overweight and even obese people often eat far less than their thin counterparts. Many arguments have been advanced to try to explain this discrepancy, but none are convincing. (We'll review some of these theories in Chapter 4.) Most of us have personally known at least one or two *under*weight individuals who have been unsuccessful at gaining, no matter how many calories they consumed. Furthermore, the theory of calorie requirements does not help to explain such problems as bulimia, where a person may consume as many as 15,000 calories at a sitting one day, and as little as 300 or 400 the next.

What is needed is to recover the understanding that past dietary and natural medicine traditions held: each food is different, and each has its own unique effects on the human experience. This brings us to the final point of dietary principles.

7. The Natural and Energetic Order of Diet ————

When scientists speak of "food energy," they are generally referring only to the amount of *heat* produced when the food is destroyed, or burned. This is measured as calories; *calorie* literally means "heat." However, this is only one aspect of energy, and it describes only what is directly measurable as a food is destroyed.

When we speak of a food's energetic character, we mean something far different. Every food, every life from, has its own unique set of attributes and behavior, which might be called its "life energy." These energetic qualities are created by how the food grew or how it was formed, in what kind of environment it lives, and many other factors. For example, a cow and a human being think, move, and behave very differently. It should come as no surprise that very different behavior and physical attributes are produced in children drinking cow's milk and those given human mother's milk. In understanding how foods will affect us, we need to have a way to perceive their overall character, their energetic behavior.

The broadest example is to compare animal and vegetable foods. We already know that the animal and plant kingdoms are very different; in fact, in many ways they are mirror images of each other. Plants, for instance, grow their roots down and out into the soil to gather nutrients, while we carry our "roots" internally in the small intestine where our nutrients are absorbed. (The intestinal flora we described earlier are quite similar to microbes in the soil that assist in the nourishment of plant roots.) The plant's respiratory system develops as leaves, expanding up and outward, while our lungs develop inward into a dense, com-pacted form. Further, the plant's leaf system inhales carbon dioxide and exhales oxygen, while our lungs do the reverse.

While plants are stationary, we are mobile. We are made largely of protein, and store our excess calories largely in the form of fat; plants are made primarily of carbohydrate, and store their energies as carbohydrate (especially complex carbohydrate) and as oils.

Thus, animals and plants are dominated by opposite, balancing forces, which we can call *yin* and *yang*. Yin, representing a more passive, quiet and expanding tendency, is more characteristic of the vegetable kingdom. Yang, a more active and contracting tendency, describes the structure and behavior more of the animal kingdom. This kind of comparison can be drawn between many other contrasting pairs of food types. And indeed, the comparing of yin and yang traits can be extended to features within the human body and metabolism, to aspects of human behavior, and in fact to all phenomena in the world.

Fig. 5 The Opposite Characteristics—Yin and Yang—of Plants and the Human Body

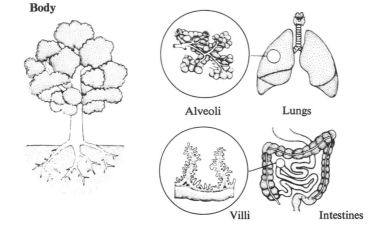

Alveoli   Lungs

Villi   Intestines

The leaves of the tree—expanded, yin structures—breathe in carbon dioxide (CO_2) and give out oxygen (O_2), while human lungs—compacted, yang structures—breathe in oxygen and give out carbon dioxide. Roots absorb liquid nourishment from the soil in the case of plants, while in the case of human beings, intestinal villi, which have an inverse structure, absorb the nourishment of food molecules. Many other opposite characteristics can be observed in the structures and functions of plants and the human body.

serve as an introduction to this simple yet profoundly comprehensive way of looking at the world.

The exchange of gasses between plants and animals is typical of the complementing relationship of such opposites. Other examples include the attraction of positive and negative electrical poles, or the dynamic balance we naturally seek between periods of mental and physical activity, or of activity and rest—or for that matter, between using our left arm and right arm, or arms and legs. Like the turning of the tides and seasons, all events in nature strive for harmony by balancing their relative degrees of yin and yang qualities.

The axiom "you are what you eat" can be more easily understood in terms of yin and yang. Consuming animal foods such as meat or poultry, produces a strong yang effect in our body. For example, our blood sugar level may tend to decrease more easily, our internal organs contract and become tighter, our skin may become drier, and we tend to feel harder and less flexible overall. In terms of behavior, we tend to grow more focused, willful, and aggressive, more active, and more preoccupied with Figure 6 illustrates some common examples of yin and yang, and will the material world and immediate circumstances. These are all more yang characteristics.

Fig. 6   Examples of Yin and Yang

	Yin ▽*	Yang △*
Attribute	Centrifugal force	Centripetal force
Tendency	Expansion	Contraction
Function	Diffusion	Fusion
	Dispersion	Assimilation
	Separation	Gathering
	Decomposition	Organization
Movement	More inactive, slower	More active, faster
Vibration	Shorter wave and higher frequency	Longer wave and lower frequency
Direction	Ascent and vertical	Descent and horizontal
Position	More outward and peripheral	More inward and central
Weight	Lighter	Heavier
Temperature	Colder	Hotter
Light	Darker	Brighter
Humidity	Wetter	Drier
Density	Thinner	Thicker
Size	Larger	Smaller
Shape	More expansive and fragile	More contractive and harder
Form	Longer	Shorter
Texture	Softer	Harder
Atomic particle	Electron	Proton
Elements	N, O, P, Ca, etc.	H, C, Na, As, Mg, etc.
Environment	Vibration . . . Air . . . Water . . . Earth	
Climatic effects	Tropical climate	Colder climate
Biological	More vegetable quality	More animal quality
Sex	Female	Male
Organ structure	More hollow and expansive	More compacted and condensed
Nerves	More peripheral, orthosympathetic	More central, parasympathetic
Attitude, emotion	More gentle, negative, defensive	More active, positive, aggressive
Work	More psychological and mental	More physical and social
Consciousness	More universal	More specific
Mental function	Dealing more with the future	Dealing more with the past
Culture	More spiritually oriented	More materially oriented
Dimension	Space	Time

* For convenience, the symbols ▽ for Yin, and △ for Yang are used.

By contrast, a completely vegetarian diet will tend to relax these yang traits, making our body softer and our mind more quiet, calm, and peaceful. A diet composed of more extremely yin foods, such as fruits, sugar, milk, and frequent raw salads, produces more strongly yin effects. Our organs may grow weak and underactive, our blood sugar level may

43

tend to rise too high, our tissues and muscles may lose tone, and we may be more prone to infection. In our behavior, we will tend to become overly passive or shy, disorganized, lacking in discipline, and more preoccupied with the psychological or spiritual worlds and more distant, theoretical or abstract concerns.

Fig. 7   General Yin (▽) and Yang (△) Categorization of Foods

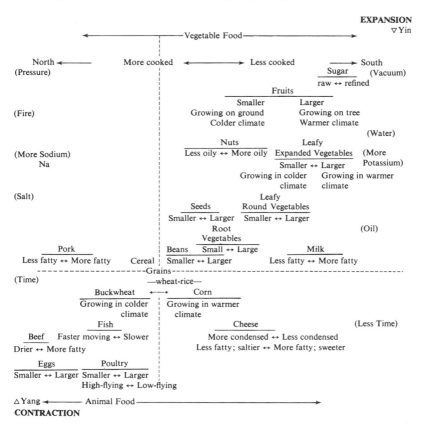

The above chart gives the general classification of food groups from yang to yin. However, more precise classification should be made upon examination of environmental conditions, nature and structure, chemical compounds, and effect upon our physical and mental conditions. Also, cooking can greatly change food qualities from yin to yang and yang to yin.

In terms of human diet and health, this suggests that our diet should naturally seek to strike a dynamic balance between more yin foods and more yang foods. This, in fact, is just what we are doing when we get thirsty for beer or water after eating something salty: salt is strongly yang and contracting, while water is expansive and yin, and alcohol even more so. A quick glance at Figure 7 reveals that consuming more yang foods leads automatically to a desire for more yin foods. This has resulted in such commonplace pairings as steak and ice cream, eggs and orange juice, or cheese and wine.

However, a diet based on such extremes, while it strikes a "balance" of a sort, does so through extreme fluctuations in our metabolism, and this exacts a toll on our health. Learning to use the principles of yin and yang more consciously allows us to select foods with more mild, moderate tendencies. This, in turn, is easier to balance, and places less wear and tear on the body and psyche.

When studying Figure 7, please remember that this represents only a general, simplified spectrum for the purpose of illustrating the principle of yin and yang in food. Each food actually has its own unique balance of both yin and yang traits (though one force or the other always predominates), and this balance is also affected to some degree by the way a food is prepared. The serious student of yin and yang can learn a great deal more through other books devoted to this subject,[11] as well as through macrobiotic lectures and cooking classes, which are available in most areas throughout the United States.

So that we can begin to understand the relationship of food and our behavior in more detail, Figure 8 presents a summary of the types of thinking often produced by extremes of yin and yang in diet. This is organized into seven stages of progressively more yin attitudes, and seven stages of increasingly yang extremes of thought. Either tendency, when carried to the extreme, can eventually lead to severe mental disorders, revealing a sense of complete separation from the reality of the universe around us.

Fig. 8 Development of Yin and Yang Mental Imbalances

Yin Cause
Overconsumption of sugar and other sweeteners, fruits and juices, dairy products, hot spices, some vegetables of tropical or semi-tropical origin, chemicals, most medications, drugs, alcohol, ex-

Yang Cause
Overconsumption of meat, eggs, poultry and other animal foods, fish (especially red-meat and blue-skinned fish or smoked or salt-cured fish), excessive salt, baked and burned foods. Also, lack of

cessive liquids. Also, lack of good quality minerals and other mildly yang foods.

sufficient liquid intake, vegetables and other mildly yin foods.

1) General mental fatigue, manifesting as a complaining attitude and gradual loss of clarity in thinking and behavior.

General mental fatigue, manifesting as harshness, abrupt changes of mind and gradual loss of steadiness in thinking and behavior.

2) Feeling of melancholy, timidity, gradual loss of ambition and confidence; the beginning of forgetfulness and confusion.

Beginning of rigidity, gradually developing into stubbornness and insistent attention to trivial matters.

3) Anxiety, irritability and fear, prevailing depression, persistently defensive attitude.

Excitability, short temper, prevailing discontentment, persistently offensive attitude.

4) Deep suspicion and skepticism, misinterpretation and misconceptions, general retreating attitude.

Overconfidence and pride, rigid conceptualization, producing various "isms" and beliefs.

5) Discrimination and prejudice based on feelings of inferiority.

Discrimination and prejudice based on feelings of superiority.

6) Loss of self-discipline; chaos in thinking, attitude and behavior; schizophrenic symptoms.

Loss of self-reflection; egocentric thinking, attitude and behavior; paranoid symptoms.

7) Yin arrogance: total inability and refusal to adapt to the environment, including other people and ideas; suffering from the delusion that "I am the victim of the world."

Yang arrogance: total inability and refusal to accept the environment, including other people and ideas; suffering from the delusion that "I am the complete master of the world."

---

1 For a detailed discussion of carbohydrate metabolism, please refer to the authors' *Diabetes and Hypoglycemia.*

2 Trowell p. 15.

3 *Diet and Nutrition: A Holistic Approach*, Dr. Rudolph Ballentine, p. 283–285.

4 Ballantine, p. 121.

5 In fact, the recent decline in dairy and meat consumption in the U.S. has contributed to the massive economic upheaval in modern mid-Western farms, as we begin shifting back in the direction of more traditional eating patterns.

46

6 *Excessive Eating*, Slochoner, J.A., Human Science Press, Inc., NY 1983.

7 *Dietary Goals*, p. 53.

8 See *Obesity, Weight Loss, and Eating Disorders* in the Macrobiotic Food and Cooking Series.

9 P. 90 ff.

10 "Topics in Primary Care Medicine: Approach to Obese Patients," Eugene V. Boisaubin, MD; *The Journal of Western Medicine*, May 1984.

11 See particularly *The Macrobiotic Diet, The Book of Macrobiotics, Macrobiotic Cooking For Everyone*, and *Macrobiotic Home Remedies*.

12 Adapted from *The Book of Macrobiotics*, pp. 136–7.

3. The Origin of Hunger ━━━━━━━━━

The questions, What is hunger? And what exactly causes it? are central to the entire issue of eating disorders. It would seem obvious that hunger is simply an instinct, coming from the awareness that we need nourishment to continue existing. And it may be that in various animals this is basically so. But at least for human beings, the issue is not so simple.

There are quite a few theories concerning hunger. Psychological explanations of hunger were particularly popular in the nineteenth century, with the advent of the Freudian and other schools of psychoanalysis. In the early days of this century, many scientists focused on the possible hormonal causes of hunger and satiety. The past several years have seen a great deal of new research in the field of *neurochemistry*, much of it oriented around the question of hunger.

Some theories are advanced to describe the psychological processes, social conditioning, or hereditary features that may control our desire for food. Others attempt to explain the *mechanisms* of hunger, that is, how the information that we are low on nourishment travels through the body and reaches the level of conscious awareness.

One such route may be the *vagus nerve*, which is the central nerve controlling the autonomic nervous system. (The *autonomic nervous system* controls body functions without our conscious awareness; its opposite is the *central nervous system*, which includes our senses and conscious thought centers.) When food reaches the stomach, *peptides* are released and enter the blood; they are detected by the vagus nerve, which sends electrical messages to the brain. These messages eventually reach the *hypothalamus*, deep inside the brain, which is thought to be the general control center for impulses such as hunger. Finally, the hypothalamus interprets this information as meaning we are full, and "turns off" the hunger impulse. One confirmation of this theory is that when the vagus nerve is severed in experimental animals they continue eating long after their needs are met, sometimes even until the point of literally bursting.[1]

On the other hand, neurophysiology also tells us that the stomach is stimulated to begin secreting its digestive fluids when we simply smell or look at an attractive food. Beginning from our senses and the conscious regions of the brain, messages are being sent through the reverse pathway, presumably, through the hypothalamus and vagus nerve to the stomach itself. This poses an interesting question: does the stomach control the brain, or vice versa? Which is the *real* source of the "hunger impulse"?

The problem with such theories is that they show what *may* happen in certain circumstances, but they do not satisfactorily explain whether this is always so, sometimes so, or only occasionally so. It is obvious that the majority of our population frequently eats beyond the point of nutritional need. But can we assume, because of this, that the vagus nerve or hypothalamus has been impaired in such cases?

Another theory suggests that the liver is the "first organ to know" when we are eating. The liver and pancreas control secretions of various hormones, most notably *insulin*. When insulin is released into the blood, it causes "free" glucose, fatty acids, and amino acids in the blood either to be burned away or to clump together in "bound" form, as *glycogen* (a storage form of glucose), fat, or protein. The hypothalamus, however, also has insulin receptors. According to this theory, the levels of insulin in the bloodstream (controlled by the liver and pancreas) may be "telling" our hypothalamus when we are hungry, when we are full, and even how fat or lean we are.

We will look at some of these theories in Chapter 4. Overall, though, there is little agreement as to what are the most important factors or central mechanisms governing hunger. Certainly, there must be *many* physiological and psychological mechanisms involved, but no comprehensive framework has been suggested to unify the various points of view. Here again, to understand the essential nature of hunger, the broader perspective provided by macrobiotic thinking is sorely needed. Attempting to conduct this inquiry while lacking such a large view is comparable to investigating why Da Vinci painted the Mona Lisa, and who it truly represents, by analyzing the chemical contents of the paint used!

The Universal Nature of Hunger

The Gospel According to Thomas is a recently discovered manuscript containing teachings attributed to Jesus. While this attribution is still a matter of some scholarly controversy, the simple language of the recorded conversations between master and students contains a wealth of insight into the workings of God, nature, and the universe.

One such saying is given in response to the disciples questioning about the Kingdom of Heaven: "When you make the two one, and when you make the inner as the outer and the outer as the inner, and when you make the male and the female into a single one . . . then shall you enter [the Kingdom]."[2]

We can say this in different words: harmonizing opposites, and uniting apparently contrasting forces or phenomena into a balanced unity, is the key to our realizing our oneness with the universe.

The Bible itself contains myriad references to the image of harmonizing opposites. The passage from Isaiah describing the coming of an ideal world is perhaps the most well-known: "The wolf shall dwell with the lamb, and the leopard shall lie down with the kid . . . and the cow and the bear shall feed . . . and the lion shall eat straw like an ox."[3] In many passages, the nature of God is expressed as "alpha and omega" or "the first and the last"; and the human condition, that is, the state of seeking for such balance or yearning for this universal, spiritual fulfillment, is often expressed with the images of hunger and thirst. These expressions reveal a profound understanding of the origin and true nature of hunger. And though many of these images have been incorporated into our everyday speech, few reflect on their full implications.

Yin and Yang

As we have discussed, the universe is animated by the constant interplay of yin and yang. The more opposite two things are, the more they will tend to attract each other. And they will continue being thus attracted until their nature changes, or until they finally merge with one another and cancel out each other's opposite qualities. Depending on the nature of the interaction, this may produce a peaceful or stable quality, or it may result in a powerful new force of movement.

For example, iron and oxygen are respectively more yang and more yin, and are therefore strongly attracted together. When they merge they may produce rust; if this takes place in the context of our blood—the iron at the center of our hemoglobin meeting with oxygen inhaled through our lungs—our blood cells become red. Sodium is still more yang than iron, so its attraction to oxygen is even stronger. If they are brought together in a laboratory, an explosion is the result.

The attraction of oxygen and hydrogen is another example. These two atoms are so nearly equivalent in their yin and yang natures that when they merge the result—water—has an extraordinarily neutral quality. This finely balanced nature has earned water the title of "universal solvent," and is the reason that three-fourths of the earth's surface and the major portion of biological organisms are composed of water.

Between the two sexes, the male gender is more yang, and the female is more yin. The dynamic this polarity produces manifests on the most basic level, obviously, as sexual attraction. And when this attraction is fulfilled by the merging of sex, the result may include a very peaceful feeling and, sometimes, the beginning of a new life.

On a physiological and chemical level, the polarity of yin and yang affects our appetite in many ways. Within the world of biological life, the central polarity is that between the animal and vegetable kingdoms. On an immediate level, this is the basis of our natural sense of hunger—our innate desire to absorb food is not fundamentally different from the attraction of one sex to another, or of oxygen to hydrogen.

Beyond the plant world a larger polarity exists. This is the natural impulse to bridge the gap between the *animate* and *inanimate* worlds, in other words, the attraction of *both* plants and animals to water, minerals, air, and other elements of the environment. Our sense of need for both air and water is greater than our drive for solid foods. Still greater than our attraction to the elements of our *material* environment, is our attraction to our *energetic* or *spiritual* environment.

Overall, the central polarity of our lives could be summed up as the difference between "me" and the rest of the world. Actually, as we saw in Chapter 1, this is not an absolute separation. The boundary lines between a person and his environment are really no more than points of reference, like the point at which day "changes into" night, or the hollow interior of the small intestine's villi where food becomes part of our bloodstream.

Yet, though the distinction of these boundaries is not an absolute one, it does exist. And our greatest desire, actually our *only* desire, is to transcend these boundaries, dissolve our sense of separation, and feel ourselves merge once again with the environment that brought us into existence. This is the origin of hunger; it could be called our "Life Hunger." All our relative desires reflect this basic, universal source.

On an immediate biological level, we feel this through the urge to eat and drink. The physiological mechanisms through which we sense our capacities at the moment—when we can follow through with this desire, and when we have reached a temporary balance point—are simply examples of the way our body and psyche interpret this universal attraction.

On other levels, we see it in an infant's grasping for sensory experience, and in the innate curiosity of the child. It manifests in the desire to travel, to extend our senses out through physical space, and in the thirst for knowledge, even in the spiritual quest to penetrate the underlying significance of our lives.

Of course, we do not begin acting on all these levels immediately upon birth. In the natural growth of a human being, the many layers of Life Hunger tend to unfold gradually, beginning on the most immediate levels, and proceeding in an orderly manner to larger and larger levels. This is dictated by our awareness, which tends to grow in seven levels often described in macrobiotic thought as the *Seven Levels of Judgement*. These are described below.

The Seven Levels of Judgement ━━━━━━━━━━━━━━

1. *The Mechanical Level.* Beginning well before birth, we learn to interpret, coordinate, and balance the alternating currents of our own nervous impulses. An example of this level is the development of the nursing impulse in a newborn. This level generally operates below the threshold of consciousness, and manages the functions of our body organs and muscular activities.

2. *The Sensorial Level.* Again beginning before birth, this level of awareness is our primary focus of concentration during our first months after birth. This includes our learning to distinguish between yin and yang as perceived through our senses, such as the sense of hot and cold, dark and light and various colors, different sounds and their implications.

3. *The Emotional Level.* As we begin to master the basics of our body mechanics and senses, particularly with the development of crawling, the next level gradually absorbs our greatest concentration. We grow aware of our own reactions to the events in our lives, and first become truly aware of "ourselves," in the sense of having a conscious identity as separate from the world around us. We learn to distinguish more acutely between the character and attitudes of different people around us, and refine and differentiate between our own emotional states. Over time and repeating experiences, we begin to realize that periods of despair or loss (such as when our mother leaves the room for a few moments) will be followed by times of fun and gaiety. Patience and a deeper sense of time begin to arise. A fascination with patterns of experience gives rise to the faculties of conscious recognition and memory. Random repetition gives way to an appreciation of games, and with it, a sense of humor. Though this development precedes formal language, we begin to express ourselves in conscious patterns of sound and gesture.

4. *The Logical or Intellectual Level.* Most clearly seen with the development of formal language, our awareness of the patterns of change begins to extend beyond our immediate experience. Our sense of both time and space enlarges dramatically, and we start to perceive the mechanics of the universe as rational processes even outside the realm of our senses or feelings. While this sphere of awareness does not carry the immediate impact of sensory or emotional experience, the sheer range within which it can operate often makes it a thrilling discovery. (Many people find this sphere so entrancing that they may

be unable or unwilling to progress further for many years.)

5. *The Social or Sociological Level.* While the fourth level of judgement extends our awareness in time and space, this fifth level can be described as increasing the *depth* of our awareness. We begin to penetrate deeper into the meanings of things our logical minds have explained. A deeper understanding of the cycles of change and human experience begin to develop here, sometimes leading to a clearer sense of economy, ecology, and social justice. This level also describes the deepening of *spiritual* vision, as we begin more directly to sense the energy and spirit underlying physical phenomena. This also brings about a more direct sense and respect for the world of nature, not as objects of sensory description, emotional reaction, or logical calculation, but as fellow existences in the spiral of creation.

6. *The Philosophical or Ideological Level.* Nowadays when people speak of "ideology" they are generally referring to economic theory, such as socialism or capitalism. We would describe these more as sociological or intellectual theories (depending upon the depth of their view—when they are merely repetitions of ideas others have already developed, this would be described more accurately as *mechanical* awareness!). In this context, ideological judgement refers to the natural outgrowth of the previous level. Our observations of the meaning behind events leads us to sense the rhythm of life itself. This is the point at which we truly begin to understand, not as intellectual knowledge but as a constant, direct reality, that all seeming antagonisms are actually complementary. For example, we no longer see unhappiness as "bad" and happiness as "good," but realize and accept that they are two aspects of the same rhythm of human emotion. A deep sense of justice arises with this level of awareness; the great religions and philosophies of human history have arisen from philosophical judgement.

7. *The Absolute or Comprehensive Level.* With the full unfolding of the human capacity for understanding, the knowledge of yin and yang, the rhythm of life, becomes an automatic part of our lives, and we operate more from the level of accurate *intuition* than from consciously applied thought. With this level, we find that we feel free to act according to any and all other levels of judgement at will, depending on what we intuitively feel is appropriate at the moment. For example, a person who is living with this scope of awareness may sometimes appear to be a saint, and at other times suddenly

show anger or profound sentimental indulgence. The life of such a person is expressed as one who is constantly experiencing balance and always living fully in the moment, while at the same time aware of its broadest implications in space and time.

Our appetite for life manifests in very different ways, depending upon which level of judgement is most prominent. Further, the act of choosing and eating solid food itself carries different meanings to us, according to the principal focus of our judgement. Let us see how these seven levels apply to our eating habits.

The Seven Levels of Eating

1. *Eating According to the Mechanical Level.* The mechanical level refers to eating automatically to follow our appetite, without using any clear consciousness. At this level, we eat without regard to reason, choice, or preference, eating whatever is at hand, whenever the mechanical impulse arises. Another expression of this level is the choosing of foods according to what is at the closest grocery store, or what is selling at the cheapest price. This way of eating tends to nourish a way of living that responds spontaneously, with no thought or idea, to external stimuli.

2. *Eating According to the Sensorial Level.* On the sensorial level, our food choices are dictated by how foods taste, smell, look, and feel. The physical act of eating is more important to us than what effects the food has after we have eaten it. Exaggeration of this level can lead to using food as gratification or indulgence, and to blindly following popular tastes. Eating from this level tends to nourish a way of living driven by the goals of sensory pleasure and material satisfaction.

   The overwhelming majority of food choices in modern society are dictated by the first two levels of judgement alone. This is evident by observing the way foods are advertised.

3. *Eating According to the Emotional Level.* Eating on the emotional level implies food choices based on what makes us feel good, though not necessarily in a sensory way. For example, eating the foods we enjoyed as a child, or preferring a variety of favorites from certain periods of our lives when we felt we were happiest. Another aspect of this level more directly concerns foods' actual effects on us. Certain foods often have a specific effect on our mood, and we may eat them consistently in order to achieve that emotional result.

Alcohol, for example, may lead us to feel we have overcome inhibitions. Refined sugar can make us feel "clever" or even giddy; a morning cup of coffee can "take the edge off" our surly mood. Though many are not consciously aware of it, dairy products can make us feel taken care of. For many poor people, particularly those who experienced deprivation in less modernized countries in their youth, white bread or white rice makes them feel wealthy. If we are living our lives with our primary focus on our emotions, these effects and associations can become addictive. Eating from this level tends to nourish an intellectually more limited, even childish way of life, in which we are driven by our moods and sentiments.

4. *Eating According to the Intellectual Level.* The intellectual level is the level of reason and systematized thinking. Modern nutritional theory is based squarely on this sphere of thought, analyzing the foods we eat in terms of scientific concepts based upon controlled experiments. The greatest limitation of this perspective is that it often excludes consideration of the environment. For example, we may decide to supplement a diet of animal products and refined foods with prepared vitamins and minerals, without asking ourselves larger questions such as, Can the environment easily support this approach to eating? or, Is this really the way I am naturally designed to eat? This is also the level of rationalization. Explanations of our eating habits from this level are often offered (to others or to ourselves) to justify actions which may actually be dictated by more immediate impulses. We often eat foods simply because we are familiar with them, or prefer the way they taste, and clothe our choice in a rational explanation.

5. *Eating According to the Sociological Level.* Eating according to the sociological level is an approach to diet based on a social conscience, guided by ideas of fair distribution and social equality. A sense of ethics, morals, and economic consciousness may suggest the appropriate types and volumes to be consumed. Governmental policies often administer food programs from this economic level of thinking. The awareness of the environment also enters here, considering which patterns of eating make the wisest use of the earth's resources. Another example would be an individual's choice to eat less as a gesture of empathy with starvation in other areas, or to avoid certain foods because of the political or economic conditions under which they are grown or produced.

6. *Eating According to the Philosophical Level.* The philosophical level of eating is based upon a deeper understanding of man and nature. We may choose or avoid certain foods out of our understanding of the role they play in the design of life itself. We also select our foods and control the way they are prepared and eaten with an awareness of the effects they will have on our spiritual consciousness. The great dietary teachings of Judaism, Hinduism, Buddhism, Taoism, and Shintoism are examples of this level of eating. Using a deep comprehension of yin and yang to choose our foods macrobiotically also stems from this awareness. However, it should be noted that simply following the dictates of established traditions, or blindly following another's interpretation of yin and yang without developing our own personal understanding, does not occupy the sixth level of judgement, but more accurately the first, or mechanical level.

7. *Eating According to the Comprehensive Level.* Eating according to the comprehensive level could also be described as eating according to free consciousness, or by following unerringly clear intuition. With a lucid understanding of all the other approaches to food, a person of this level uses no special approach or system, but automatically chooses, prepares and eats a variety of foods according to the situation, creating a masterpiece of balance in any circumstance. This level also expresses itself as eating in such a way as to realize one's greatest dream.

While this last level may seem highly idealized or unattainable, this is not exactly the case. While few of us have mastered the first six spheres of judgement, *everyone* exercises the seventh level of judgement to some degree, even if only for momentary periods and without being fully aware of it. It is not difficult to reach this level; in a sense, everyone already experiences it partially. The challenge of human judgement is to develop our consciousness through all the first six levels, one by one, achieving a deeply practical understanding of each in turn. This creates the foundation for graduating from the world of relative likes and dislikes, beliefs and disbeliefs, and finally exercising our judgement as the truly free creatures we are designed to be. This is the goal of macrobiotics.

Whether or not we follow this natural progression smoothly depends on the question of balance. If we are not able to find a satisfactory balance of opposites while focusing on one level, it becomes more difficult to pursue the next level clearly. For example, if our food is overly rich, laden with butter, spices, and refined sweeteners, our senses are overstimulated and it is very difficult to achieve a feeling of stability in our sensory judgement. As we grow to overemphasize our senses and give our attention to the pursuit of strong cravings, it is very difficult to develop our emotional perspective along balanced lines. Likewise, an overemphasis on our emotional satisfaction or an emotionally under- or over-nourished condition makes keen thinking and clear decision-making a problem.

Though the higher levels of judgement may have a great appeal because they seem loftier, the first level of judgement is actually the most crucial. Our mechanical, physiological, unconsciously controlled sense of stability and balance is the foundation upon which all conscious judgement rests. And our ability to harmonize this internal condition is most directly affected by our food. This is why macrobiotic thinking considers everyday diet as the most crucial factor affecting our thinking, judgement, and human experience. It is not that diet is the *only* factor, but it is the most basic.

To sum up, hunger for food is one manifestation of our hunger for life itself, which is our natural desire to merge ourselves with the environment that gave us birth. This Life Hunger animates our entire existence, and is exercised in increasing dimensions as our judgement and awareness unfolds. While this judgement embraces the highest forms of human expression, it is based most fundamentally upon our internal condition, which stems most centrally from our diet. Imbalance on this primary level will manifest as imbalances in every other sphere of our human experience.

In instances of eating disorders, something has gone awry in our relationship to our world; we are unable to interpret this Life Hunger in ways that lead us toward a greater life. The number of calories we consume, or the number of pounds our frames carry, may be the most obvious outward signs of the problem—but it is clear that we have somehow more deeply altered our sense of balance.

---

[1] One cannot help but wonder at the mentality of research that finds it necessary to torture animals in order to understand people.

[2] *The Gospel of Thomas*, trans. Guillaumont et al., Harper & Row, 1959, p. 17 ff.

[3] The Book of Isaiah, 11: 6–7.

4. Overweight and Obesity ▬▬▬▬▬

Overweight has proved to be a difficult term to define precisely. Technically speaking, obesity means being 20 percent over the "ideal weight" for one's height; *overweight* simply describes the weight range between "ideal" and "obese."

These definitions illustrate the slippery nature of the problem. Just what is the "ideal weight" for a certain height? The figures in general use come from a chart compiled by the Metropolitan Life Insurance Company, for decades considered the experts on what individuals should weigh. Metropolitan's chart reflects extensive statistics gathered from over four million Americans, correlating weight to longevity. In other words, they tell us at what average weights Americans are currently living the longest. Unfortunately, they tell us nothing whatsoever about whether people of these specific weights are healthy or sick, happy or miserable.

Research data gathered by diabetes specialists tell us that virtually 100 percent of American nursing home residents suffer from some degree of diabetes.[1] Nearly 97 percent of Americans over the age of sixty have arthritic conditions progressed enough to appear on an X-ray.[2] If our grandmother is currently living in a nursing home, crippled with arthritis, taking handfuls of aspirin or other anti-inflammatory drugs for the pain, as well as medications for high blood sugar, Metropolitan Life will still take her weight into account as "ideal," simply because she is alive. They do not consider whether she might be far happier and healthier if she ate differently and weighed a different numbers of pounds.

Several years ago Metropolitan Life caused a stir by raising these figures for the first time since 1959. This news was most likely hailed with relief by the majority of Americans who heard about it. A *Time* magazine story on the change began, "Dieters ate their desserts with a little less guilt last week," and many health professionals expressed enthusiasm.[3] A renowned nutrition expert from Harvard University explained his support of the new standards: "Fighting Mother Nature [that is, the attempt to lose weight] is getting to be a serious problem."

Yet quite a few authorities criticized the new figures. In the same *Time* article, Dr. Virgil Brown, chairman of the American Heart Association, explained, "The fact that fatter people are living longer may merely reflect the growing success of medical intervention in weight-related ailments." This is essentially another way of describing the situation of diabetic nursing home residents given above.

While for many it is tempting to interpret the new 1983 policy to mean that a weight that was obese in 1982 became only six or seven pounds overweight in 1983, the opposite is more likely the case. The upward crawl of our standard of measurement simply shows that as our average weight climbs higher and higher, we are accommodating our national condition by adjusting upwards our vision of what is "normal"!

Overweight versus Overfat ─────────────

Another problem with the usual weight standards is that while they measure how many pounds we weigh, they do not tell us anything about the *quality* of our weight. Let us consider two adult men of the same general skeletal build, each weighing 140 pounds. The first man may be carrying 32 pounds of fat, while the second may have only 21 pounds of fat on his body and 11 more pounds of muscle mass. If we judge them sheerly on the basis of the bathroom scale, they would be considered "identical," and neither might be judged as overweight. In fact, the first would be considerably over*fat*, while the second would probably be in much better condition.

Measuring the percentage of the body consisting of fat is a far more accurate indicator of health than total body weight. This is accomplished by a procedure known as the *underwater immersion test*, based on the fact that fat floats while lean muscle and bone (called *Lean Body Mass*) does not. Performing this procedure with accuracy requires some fairly sophisticated equipment, but we can get a general estimate of our Lean Body Mass and fat percentage just by floating in a lake or pool and gradually emptying our lungs. At above 25 percent fat, we will float easily; at 12 percent , just half that fat percentage, we will readily sink.[4]

According to fitness specialist Covert Bailey, the maximum fat percentages for good health are about 15 percent for men and 22 percent for women. More active people may easily have less—a slim cross-country runner may have as little as 6 percent body fat.[5] In general, the less the percentage of body fat, the more efficiently our metabolism operates and the better the health we enjoy. (Obviously, this statement does not apply to cases of extreme underweight.) In his popular book *Fit or Fat*, Bailey states, "We have measured thousands of people, however, and most men seem to average 23 percent fat, most women 36 percent . . . If you are only 5 pounds overweight, it is probable that you are at least 13 pounds overfat."[6]

Even using the Metropolitan Life figures, it is estimated that over

50 percent of Americans are overweight. In view of the shortcomings of using this standard, it seems likely that a much higher proportion of the population is overweight, overfat, or fat.

Contradictions and Controversies ━━━━━━━━━

As mentioned earlier, the field of weight and appetite research is riddled with opposing points of view. In her widely respected book, *Eating Disorders*, Dr. Hilde Bruch describes the prevailing confusion in obesity and anorexia research:

> . . . The majority of papers continue to focus on one or other aspects as the 'cause' of the condition. The more an investigator is convinced of the importance of his own theory, the more he is inclined to use his particular findings as [an] explanation for the whole picture.[7]

The same can be said of entire eras of scientific focus. Though there are many interweaving threads of various approaches to overweight, certain types of theories have emerged as the primary focus during periods of history when their particular scientific field developed. To put it simply, opinions as to the "real cause" of overweight have seemed to follow the prevailing scientific fashion.

Thus, the *psychoanalytical* approach of Freud and his colleagues supported various psychological views in the last century. Darwin's theory of "survival of the fittest" led to *hereditary* and *evolutionary* theories of weight control. These opposing perspectives clashed in the famous "hereditary versus environment" debate, which is still active today. The growing field of *endocrinology* in the early decades of this century led many to advance differing hypotheses of a hormonal cause of overweight.

Advances in technology issuing from research programs during World War II resulted in greater accuracy in the observation and measurement of many physiological functions. This technical sophistication has made possible a variety of *metabolic* theories, which have revamped some of the older and more simplistic models of endocrinology and refined them to explain the newer observations. Within the past few years this direction has moved further with the almost explosive growth of research in *neurochemistry*.

Meanwhile, the older psychoanalytical models have begun to give way in some circles to more updated versions of behavioral and transactional psychology. These modern approaches have to some degree grown out of "systems" theory and computer science. Generally, they deal less with Freud's broadly generalized assumptions, such as the universal potency of primitive instincts and the deeply symbolic significance of childhood experiences with defecation and sexuality, and explore more the behavior patterns through which individuals relate to circumstances, to others, and to their image of themselves.

Ultimately, none of these dozens of approaches have offered a comprehensive, lasting solution to this problem. Though many individuals have been helped to some degree, the majority still suffer, and their number grows each year. However, each line of scientific inquiry has made some positive contributions to our general understanding, and for these contributions we are deeply grateful.

To review all of these approaches in depth would be far beyond the scope or purpose of this book. Instead, let us look briefly at several of the most commonly cited theories, to gain an idea of the range of thought that exists on the subject, and to appreciate both their shortcomings and their contributions.

The General Framework of Overweight Theory ──────

Over the past fifty years there has been a gradual change in the general view of weight-related research. Because clinical evidence has consistently contradicted the idea that any one single theory fits every case, some of the hard lines of opinion have been obliged to soften. This has brought about a general (though not universal) recognition that a variety of factors must be operating together to cause excessive weight gain. Or at least, most researchers have begun to recognize that there are different types of cases, with perhaps one factor being more causal in some cases, and another factor carrying more weight in others.

Thus, the overall progression of general overweight theory has been a process of creating groupings. It is now less scientifically correct to speak of "an overweight problem," but rather a specific *type* of overweight problem.

The year 1900 was a landmark in this field; it saw the publication of Von Noorden's seminal book *Die Fettsucht* (literally meaning "an addiction for the accumulation of fat tissue"). Von Noorden differentiated between two main forms of obesity, which he termed *exogenous*, or "arising from the outside," and *endogenous*, "arising from the inside." Exogenous obesity meant obesity in the presence of normal metabolism, in other words, simply from eating too much, being too inactive, or both. The term endogenous (which type, interestingly, Von Noorden felt was far more rare), meant that some internal, physiological imbalance disturbing the metabolism, was creating the excess weight gain, even in the presence of normal diet and activity.

This dual classification has formed the foundation of scientific discussion on the subject. In simpler terms, we might describe these two ideas as "mind-caused overweight" and "body-caused overweight." And here we discover one of the classic errors of science: the artificial division of two things that in reality cannot be divided. Any effort to locate the source of any health problem as lying exclusively in the mind, or solely in the body, is doomed from the start. For the mind and body are two sides of one coin; neither can exist without the other, and they both are constantly changing in a dynamic balance with each other.

The mind/body classification has been further broken down into subgroups. For example, the more psychologically caused overweight has been divided into *developmental* overweight, which refers to psychological problems that develop through childhood and create deeply ingrained patterns of behavior; and *reactive* overweight, describing the tendency to overeat as a reaction to traumatic events or stressful situations, usually developing in adulthood.

The physiologically caused type of overweight can be subdivided again into two types, the first being *hereditary*, meaning that certain individuals are genetically programmed to metabolize poorly, and the second being *non-hereditary*, such as metabolic problems caused by other endocrine disorders, imbalanced nutrition, or environmental stresses.

It has also been found that there are two distinct phases of overweight. The first, the *active* or *dynamic* phase, is the period during which the excess weight is actually being gained. This is followed by the *stationary* or *stable* phase, which is the steady maintaining of the overweight condition. Some researchers feel that it is much more difficult for a subject to lose weight once the second period has begun. This brings to mind yet another grouping which has been proposed, with a variety of explanations as to its underlying causes and implications: those who can readily stick to a diet to lose weight, and those who apparently cannot.

While no truly unifying framework has yet been provided by science, these developments have begun to reveal an essential truth, which is the principle that no two things are alike.

Endocrinological and Metabolic Theories ────────

It is well known that the overweight person's metabolism of fat and sugar differs from that of a slender person's. It is estimated that obese people use energy less than 80 percent as efficiently as the non-obese. In other words, fat people tend to burn less of their food as energy, and store more of it as body fat.[8] For decades earlier in the century, it was widely held that the overweight person's "lowered metabolic rate" was due to a lack of thyroid function, even when no defect in the thyroid could actually be shown. Once more accurate measures of thyroid functions were developed, "the myth of low basal metabolism and hypothyroidism in obesity was finally laid to rest."[9]

Other endocrine and metabolic theories may be on their way to the same resting place. In recent decades, with the tremendous volume of diabetes research being conducted, increasing emphasis has been laid on the hormones of the pancreas, particularly insulin and glucagon. Insulin, as mentioned earlier, is a yang hormone that removes glucose and fatty acid molecules from the bloodstream, causing them to enter cells and be burnt as fuel or be put into storage. A number of studies have shown elevated blood insulin levels in the obese, as well as high triglyceride levels. Higher than normal insulin levels could be causing an excessive formation of triglycerides from free blood glucose. At the same time, such studies reveal diminished "carbohydrate tolerance" and "rate of carbohydrate utilization." These phrases mean that the body is not able to keep the blood's glucose levels under control, and the cells are not burning glucose properly. This is essentially a description of the early stages of diabetes.

While the theories that result from these observations differ, they are all rather vague, and often contradict one another. For example, a number of studies have excitedly announced that low glucagon levels were found in obesity. Glucagon is also termed *anti-insulin*, and essentially has insulin's reverse effects of *releasing* glucose, fatty acids, and amino acids *into* the bloodstream. Perhaps the low levels of glucagon and high levels of insulin would explain the excessive formation of fat storage. However, at least as many studies have been released showing particularly *high* glucagon levels in obese patients!

A 1979 study titled *Human Nutrition and Dietetics* concluded that although obesity "frequently accompanies hypothyroidism, hypogonadism, hypopituitarism, and Cushing's syndrome [all fairly uncommon endocrine disorders], . . . the overwhelming majority of obese patients show no evidence of endocrine disorders." Regarding the observations of altered blood levels of insulin, glucagon, glucose, and fatty acids, the report stated, "it is probable that these changes are a result of obesity and not its cause."[10]

There are other strongly held metabolic theories, notably the *thermogenesis theory* (a problem with how our body regulates the production of heat), and the set-point theory, which we will discuss shortly. These and others, however, have been contested and disproven as much as they have been championed. A 1977 report appearing in the British medical journal, *Lancet*, concluded that "there is no basis for supporting or rejecting any of the main hypotheses which have been proposed." The overall direction of this research has been growing increasingly complex, and focusing more on the detailed minutiae of physiology. In other words, it has moved further away than ever from the broad, unifying perspective that is so sorely needed. However, through its persistence and often incredible ingenuity, this avenue of research has shown science another crucial truth: all the systems of the body are thoroughly interrelated, often in marvelously intricate ways. The sheer detail of this study has begun to reveal what a delicate masterpiece of ecology the human body is. The understanding of this fact will soon lead science to a wider realization of how easily more extreme methods of therapy can upset this sensitive balance.

Psychological Theories

The possibility of obesity "being a symptom of nervous disturbance" has been discussed since before the beginning of this century. At first, the most obvious connection was that between traumatic experiences and sudden weight gain, sometimes called *reactive* obesity. One researcher has detailed four different common patterns of reactive overeating:

1. Overeating in response to general emotional tensions, such as being lonely, anxious or bored;
2. Overeating as a reaction to chronically unpleasant situations, or using food as a "substitute gratification";
3. Overeating as a symptom of a true underlying emotional illness, most commonly depression; and
4. Overeating as a result of intense, compulsive cravings that did not "seem related to external life events or emotional upheavals."[12]

The central theme of the various psychological theories is that food and the act of eating in some way becomes associated or symbolically linked in the subject's imagination with other aspects of life. Food and eating are not themselves the true problem, but since the subject is unaware of where the real problem lies, or is unable or unwilling to act on those problems, the act of eating is used as a "substitute solution."

According to Dr. Bruch, such substitution may at times do more good than harm. She cites, for example, the fact that there is one exception to the usually higher morbidity and mortality rates among the obese: their suicide rate is lower.[13] She explains this by observing that using overeating as an emotional "defense" in stressful situations may often be less destructive to the psyche than other possible ways of reacting, such as with deep despair. This view seems to be reinforced by observations of cases where a weight-loss diet is followed without any notable efforts to make positive changes elsewhere in the subject's life. In many such cases, the reduction in weight, or simply the act of following the weight-loss regime itself, seems to create more anxiety than it relieves. This has led to the conclusion that separating the underlying psychological problems from the issue of food and eating, and solving them on their own level, may often be of more importance than the actual loss of weight. (At the same time, Bruch acknowledges the physical dangers to health presented by the excess weight itself.)

As with metabolic irregularities, it is often hard to determine whether certain psychological problems play a role in causing a problem with overweight, or whether they may be a resulting effect of the psychological discomfort of being overweight in a society that despises obesity. Until several years ago, a large percentage of those attempting to treat weight problems believed psychological problems were the primary cause. Now, according to obesity authority Dr. Albert J. Stunkard, a psychiatry professor at the University of Pennsylvania, most are leaning to the theory that "these disturbances are more likely to be the results of obesity."[14]

Nevertheless, the various psychological approaches have made a positive contribution to our understanding. Perhaps the most important discovery has been that the body and mind do not operate independently, and that finding and solving underlying emotional and psychological imbalances can be a vitally important part of approaching the problem.

Genetic and Evolutionary Theories ━━━━━━━━

Hereditary theory has always held a special appeal in complex problems such as overweight, because it offers the promise of wonderfully simple explanations. Unfortunately, these explanations generally turn out to be *too* simple, and often do not fit the facts.[15] Obesity is a case in point.

There are two general observations that form the foundation for genetic theories of obesity. First, it has been found that in certain strains of laboratory animals,[16] obesity is determined by a defect in a single, identified gene. And second, obesity seems to run in families. According to some studies, the likelihood of a child of two obese parents being obese himself, as a child or as an adult, is as high as 80 percent. When only one parent is obese, the risk drops to below 10 percent.[17]

But there are considerable problems with both these points. Despite the work with laboratory rats, no such fat-determining gene has been found in humans. And though obesity seems to run in families, plausible reasons other than heredity have been suggested, including the persistence of family eating habits, exercise habits, and attitudes to food. Studies on adopted children of obese biological parents and slender adoptive parents, as well as the reverse situation, have yielded inconsistent and conflicting conclusions. The case for a genetic theory must still rely entirely on indirect evidence.

Furthermore, experience often offers a contradicting viewpoint. Dr. Bruch states that none of the severely obese, emotionally traumatized adolescents she has seen in her psyciatric practice have gone on to raise obese children, even though some had obese spouses, nor have any of these children grown into obese adults. She concludes, "I can state with . . . definiteness that whatever the transmitted genetic potential, [an obese person's] offspring are not doomed to becoming obese."[18]

A similar debate continues as to whether overweight children are more likely to become overweight adults. A 1976 paper from the Worldwatch Institute flatly declared, "Four out of five obese children become obese adults."[19] An article appearing in *Time* one decade later expressed a different viewpoint: "That notion . . . is no longer accepted. A 15-year survey of 180 infants by researchers at the University of California, Berkely, revealed that babies who were obese at six months or one year of age were most likely to be normal weight or thin by age nine."[20]

Aside from the question of direct genetic transfer from parent to child, there is a larger evolutionary view of obesity. One of the most popularly held theories is the *set-point* concept. This theory proposes that the body has some way of "setting" a predetermined ideal weight and fat content, which can be changed much like the thermostat of a central heating system. The prevalent idea is that this mechanism evolved as a means of survival during primitive times, when we presumably had often to undergo lengthy periods of fasting. In some individuals, so this theory suggests, eating large amounts tends to set this "set point" at a higher level, so that we are "preprogrammed" to keep storing more fat and burning less—that is, we program our metabolism to make us fat. This would protect us from starvation during coming times of want.

This theory, when followed through logically, leads to some interesting conclusions, such as the one presented by Dr. Eugene V. Boisaubin in the May, 1984 issue of *The Western Journal of Medicine*: "Losing weight for an obese patient may be an 'unnatural act.' "[21] One is tempted to follow this kind of circular reasoning the other way around, for example: is it then "natural" for an overly thin patient to lose still more weight?

Common sense tells us that there must be some natural system that controls our weight. However, the set-point theory, with its implied complex system of metabolic control mechanisms, has yet to be realistically explained. As the *Lancet* paper (mentioned above) states, "None of these mechanisms has been shown to exist."

The most significant contribution to our understanding provided by the proponents of the genetic theory may prove to be a negative one: through its careful scrutiny of genetic material, science may finally learn the futility of seeking for solutions in one solitary mechanism, just as medicine may learn that a lasting solution to disease is not to be found through the "Magic Bullet" approach. Concerning the evolutionary theory, it has perhaps helped keep open the door to a larger view, with its concern that the problems of modern humanity may be better understood by viewing our entire scope of historical development.

The Emerging Commonsense Perspective

Through research efforts such as these, together with the trial and error of various types of treatment they have suggested, progress has been made. The repeated failures of highly specialized approaches have virtually forced many practitioners to try and integrate their own viewpoints with others. This has sometimes occurred with a spirit of "strange bedfellows." In particular, the integration of "mind-caused" and "body-caused" approaches has often proceeded rather grudgingly. One review of various theories, with a decidedly physiological, "body-caused" orientation, admitted that "In man, at any rate, there is almost certainly some degree of cognitive control"![22] Slow as it is in coming, such recognition is certainly an encouraging development.

Features of the Emerging Commonsense Perspective

1. Overweight is not a single, uniform problem with a single, uniform solution. Although many practitioners continue to cling to one particular theory as "the" cause of overweight, and pursue one therapy as "the" important solution, most responsible approaches to overweight recognize that eating disorders are problems involving *the whole person*, and need to be approached as such. There are no "pat answers"; and further, the correct approach often needs to be tailored to each person to meet his or her particular needs.

2. Though many factors and mechanisms may be involved, they do not usually predetermine a person to overweight. While genetic factors, stressful situations, or family background may produce a *tendency* towards weight problems, such a tendency need not doom a person to obesity. Such factors can be recognized and balanced or overcome. Furthermore, many of these factors may often be *results* of an overweight condition, rather than its cause.

3. *The actual loss of weight is often not the central issue,* and in fact, often doesn't by itself result in a lasting solution. Quick-weight-loss programs, such as a high-protein, low-carbohydrate regimen or a concentrated fasting program, usually produce fast but quite temporary results. For that matter, the same thing can sometimes apply to the dietary aspect of macrobiotics, when practiced solely as an isolated dietetic technique. Eating macrobiotically in itself will, in the vast majority of cases, automatically result in a reduction of overweight and a greatly improved health condition. However, in some cases people achieve this weight loss, and then eventually return to their old eating habits. This happens because there are deeper changes that usually need to occur, beyond simply eating different foods.

4. *A sound approach to overweight should include four basic components.* Although each practitioner tends to have his own particular emphasis, whether on the psychological aspects, dietary aspects, or exercise, the mark of more responsible approaches is that they acknowledge the importance of the other aspects, and include them within their own program. These four essential aspects of approaching overweight are: 1) *balanced diet*; 2) *balanced activity* and the way we use our bodies, including exercise; 3) *balanced behavior patterns*, including emotional attitudes and psychological habits; and 4) *a balanced overall view of life*, including our view of ourselves, of food, of others, and of life itself.

The Commonsense Perspective on Balanced Diet ——

In the dietary approach to overweight, emphasis has shifted from the number of calories consumed to considering the specific types of foods used and the overall nutritional pattern. This amounts to a redefinition of priorities, from one of quantity to one of quality.

In part, this shift has arisen from observations such as Hugh Trowell's and Denis Burkitt's. In their landmark study, *Western Diseases: Their Emergence and Prevention*, Drs. Trowell and Burkitt reported findings from studying a wide range of population groups, including Inuit Eskimos, Native American groups, Australian Aborigines, different Polynesian and South African groups, and others. Their studies showed consistently that in traditional societies, obesity is normally quite rare, and occurs only to the extent that modern Western diet and lifestyle are adopted. As Trowell states in summarizing his findings, ". . . hunter-gatherers ate 'primitive food' and remained slim; modern man eats 'supermarket food' and often gets fat." He found, furthermore, that such "primitive" diets "accompanied lifelong low body weight" even when consumed in overly large volume.

Such observations suggest that it is *what* one eats, and not necessarily *how much*, that often leads to weight problems. This makes sense out of the wealth of observations that overweight people often eat significantly less than normal-weight or slim people. It also makes sense out of another widely known set of observations: in primitive and traditional cultures, obesity arises mainly in the very wealthy and powerful classes, while in modern society this pattern reverses. In affluent societies such as the United States, obesity is far more prevalent in lower classes and the economically underprivileged.[23]

The reason for this pattern reversal becomes clear when we consider what the underprivileged in affluent societies are eating. The poor peasants of an agrarian culture usually ate very little animal food or refined food, subsisting on "lowly" diets of unrefined grains and local produce. In the modern urban ghetto, the common diet consists of white bread, jam, sugary and oily snack foods, and poor quality fatty meats. Foods such as milk and cheese are freely distributed by governmental agencies. The poor of today eat the diets of yesterday's kings—and it is reflected in their girth and in their health.

In the past ten years, the value to health of "primitive" diets has also emerged in the context of such common problems as diabetes, cardiovascular disease, certain types of cancer, and allergies, to name but a few. And very fortunately, this new direction has begun to be reflected in Americans' everyday eating habits. Though this shift is still very small, it is significant. Over the past decade, the average consumption of meat, eggs, butter, lard, and sugar in the United States has respectively dropped 66 percent, 19 percent, 66 percent, 38 percent, and 23 percent. During the same period, consumption of rice increased by 60 percent, and of broccoli, by 200 percent.[24] The recent discovery by Harvard researcher Frank Sacks that many prominent fast-food chains have been using beef tallow to cook their chicken, fish, and French fries caused an immediate outcry in the news media. Such a reaction would have been unlikely ten years ago.

The new perspective also tells us that weight problems may stem as much from a *lack* of certain nutrients as from an *excess* of others. One aspect of the "primitive" diet that Trowell and Burkitt emphasize is the substantial presence of dietary fiber. *Fiber*, also called *roughage*, refers to the portion of complex carbohydrate foods that is not digested. Though popularly thought of as "bran," fiber also includes less obvious portions of such foods as unrefined grains and beans. Aside from its proven benefits in helping to regulate blood glucose and keep the digestive tract free of disease, dietary fiber is also thought to help regulate the body's internal "satiety signals," principally by letting the small intestine know when enough food has been consumed.[25] While macrobiotic eating is high in natural fiber, the modern diet of meats, dairy products, and refined foods is practically devoid of fiber.

Another common nutritional lack concerns the micronutrients found in food. In *Diet and Nutrition*, Rudolph Ballentine, M.D., states that "some of the discomfort experienced by the overweight dieter is the result of nutritional needs that are not being met . . . The restlessness and discomfort that repeatedly bring the dieter's attention back to food may also be due to a lack of vitamins and minerals."[26] A natural balance of trace minerals, for example, is necessary to properly regulate the metabolism of fats and carbohydrates, and a natural balance of B vitamins is required for the normal functioning of the intestinal tract. As with dietary fiber, modern processed foods are generally stripped of such essential micronutrients; and it is highly doubtful whether the process of artificial "enriching" or individual supplementation can recover the natural balance found in the original, unadulterated food.

A February 1986 issue of Tufts University's *Diet and Nutrition Letter* provides an example of the new commonsense approach. In a special report on weight control, it advises:

> . . . a well-balanced, low-calorie diet that provides 1,000 to 1,200 calories a day for women and several hundred more for men . . . it may come as a surprise to learn that the formula for long-term weight control has shifted away from eating protein-rich meats and cheeses and toward more complex carbohydrates—pasta, bread, cereal, and starchy vegetables. . . . for fillers, the best choices are fruits of all kinds and low-calorie vegetables including leafy greens, carrots, cauliflower, broccoli, and green beans.

The new approach follows the nutritional guidelines of *Dietary Goals*: more complex carbohydrate, less fats, less animal foods, and less processed foods. Some versions of this approach resemble macrobiotics and "primitive" diets only vaguely, while some, such as the famous Pritikin approach or the McDougall Plan, resemble macrobiotics quite closely.

A special feature of the new dietary common sense is the emphasis on breastfeeding for infants. A study of 517 children, published in June 1981 by researchers at McGill University in Montreal, provides strong evidence that breastfeeding protects against obesity, at least through adolescence. The longer the infant is nursed, the more the degree of protection seems to increase.[27] Though there have been no long-term studies to test the idea, it is assumed that this better weight regulation is a benefit of the better nutritional balance of mother's milk.[28]

Another reason may be simply that breast-fed babies tend to be overfed less than bottle-fed babies. It has long been thought that overfeeding in infancy or childhood is an important factor in adult overweight. Normally the number of fat cells in our body does not fluctuate; we usually gain weight by increasing the size of our existing fat cells, not by adding new cells. However, we do increase the number of fat cells during times of rapid overall growth, particularly the last two weeks before birth, the first two years of infancy, and the last two years before puberty.

While the average adult has about 30 to 40 billion fat cells, studies show that about three of every five obese people have added extra cells at some point. When we lose weight (or more precisely, lose fat), these cells may shrink, but they apparently do not die, even in the course of starvation; and they are always ready to take on new fat. Overfeeding in infancy (or, presumably, during the two years before puberty) can lead to the formation of extra fat cells, and an increased tendency to be overfat throughout life.

The Commonsense Perspective on Activity and Exercise

Until recently, the role of exercise in weight loss was often held in low scientific esteem. The reason for this is that most popular forms of exercise, such as swimming, sports, running, or dance, actually use an insignificant amount of calories, compared to the number most people need to lose. To lose the 3,500 to 4,000 calories that make up one pound of body fat, one would have to jog about thirty miles at an eight-mile-an-hour pace, or cycle at ten miles an hour for the equivalent of ninety miles.

With the quantity-to-quality shift in scientific thinking, though, this view has changed. Scientists have begun to realize that regular exercise produces changes in overall metabolism that may continue for as much as fifteen hours afterwards, making them far more important than the number of calories burned while actually exercising. Interestingly, properly managed exercise can also help a slightly *underweight* person to *gain* weight. It is not so much that balanced exercise causes weight *loss* per se, but rather that it helps the body learn to regulate the control of weight and the proper proportions of different types of weight.

As pointed out earlier, even people who do not appear grossly overweight often have a high body-fat percentage, with a correspondingly low percentage of muscle mass. One important feature of muscle is that it can burn fat as its fuel, while our brain and nervous system cannot. A more sedentary lifestyle is likely to use up glucose stores while under-utilizing stores of fat. Further, short bursts of activity, such as sprinting to catch a bus or running upstairs to catch a ringing phone, do not qualify as "proper exercise": they do little to burn up fat.

Keep in mind that muscles can use both glucose and fat as energy sources. The ideal proportion of these two "fuels" for muscular effort is estimated as being about 70 percent fat and 30 percent glucose. Glucose, however, will "burn" much more quickly and readily than fat. Fat is often compared to a log in a fireplace, with glucose representing the kindling. (In this analogy, refined sugar would represent gasoline or lighter fluid poured over the logs!) It normally takes more than a few minutes of the muscle's burning glucose to begin to "ignite" fat—and unless a good, high "flame" is reached, the fat may be only partially metabolized, just as a poorly ignited log will smolder and smoke.

Moreover, our muscles have different enzymes that aid in the metab-olism of glucose and fat. Between the two, the fat-burning enzymes are far more fragile, and they seem to diminish in number as the muscles' size decreases. When we rarely use our muscles vigorously, several things happen. First, the lack of muscular effort greatly reduces the amount of body fat we are using up. And what fat we do use we may be using incompletely, leaving more acid residue. Second, since muscles diminish in size when they are not used regularly, our overall percentage of muscle mass decreases, which also means losing a portion of our muscles' fat-burning enzymes. Less muscle mass and fewer enzymes means our capac-ity to utilize fat is now diminished, so our percentage of body fat will tend to increase. The more our fat-to-muscle proportion increases, the more our ability to utilize fat is diminished. In other words, the fatter we get, the more easily we will get still fatter.

The gradual loss of muscle tone through general inactivity is often accompanied by an increase in the fat content of the muscles. Typically when people lose weight without including proper physical activity as part of their program, a certain amount of weight from water and fat is lost but the muscle tone is not improved. In fact, depending upon the quality of the diet followed, the muscles may even lose additional volume of protein. Paradoxically, this is particularly true of many high protein, low carbohydrate diets, because in the absence of sufficient carbohydrate, the dietary protein is largely converted to glucose and used for energy rather than for increasing muscle mass.

In such cases, though weight has been lost, the body's ability to metabolize fat has not been improved, and may even have been dimin-ished. As soon as the program is over, the person will put weight right back on, and accumulate unused fat even more easily the second time around. This leads into the familiar "dieter's vicious cycle." Happily, the opposite process also gains momentum as a positive cycle develops. Increasing muscle tone through moderate exercise while improving dietary patterns leads to both a loss of weight *and* an increased ability of the muscles to utilize fat; over time, this cycle can lead to a recovered ability to keep weight and fat percentages in natural control.

There are additional benefits to exercise. Deeper breathing also improves overall metabolism, and exercise can physically stimulate better circulation and tone the digestive organs. Finally, being more active has a psychological benefit: it can make a person feel he is taking positive steps to change his life, which is quite true. It has been shown that obese people not only exercise less, but also use their bodies less in general, throughout the day. Even aside from specific exercise programs, simply becoming more active generally—walking short distances rather than using the car, or taking care of more domestic tasks such as house-cleaning or gardening—can be a valuable adjunct to recovery.

Finally, a word should be said about the concept of aerobics. The actual meaning of the term *aerobic exercise* is "exercise that uses air." Fat will only be metabolized properly in the presence of oxygen, so the ideal exercise is one that uses the maximum amount of oxygen. This is one reason the heart and lungs work faster during strenuous activity—to deliver more oxygen-carrying blood to the muscles.

The problem is that it is easy to drive the body to such a pace and level of strain that the rate of muscular activity exceeds our capacity to deliver sufficient oxygen to fuel it properly. When this happens, the muscles are not getting enough oxygen to operate properly. This produces strain on the muscles, and generates a greater volume of toxins which the body has to neutralize. Quite a few people are pushing themselves to their limits doing what they think is aerobic exercise, but what is actually at least partially *anaerobic* exercise.

What is aerobic for one person may not be for another. It depends on the level of activity to which our body is accustomed. A well seasoned long-distance runner may run ten miles or dance for three hours "aerobically," while for an underactive and overfat individual, simply taking a twenty minute walk may be the maximum exercise that can be accomplished without moving into the anaerobic range. For the most balanced benefits, good exercise should be followed at a moderate pace for longer periods of time, rather than at a frantic pace for shorter bursts. It is best to choose forms of exercise that involve the whole body and a variety of different types of movement, rather than one or two repetitive movements.

The Commonsense Perspective on Behavior and Psychology

In addition to eating the proper foods, reestablishing orderly eating patterns is vital. Learning to chew our food carefully, eating in regular meals rather than snacking or catching quick meals "on the run," and treating our foods with the respect we would accord our parents or grandparents, are all parts of natural diet.

As Dr. Ballentine points out in *Diet and Nutrition*, "Weight loss must be the by-product of personal evolution." An essential part of an integrated, commonsense approach to weight loss is that the person be committed to making positive overall changes in his or her life. This needs to begin with the process of honest self-reflection, where we look at our lives and see whether we are truly happy or not. We may also discover that the issue of eating has become associated in our minds with any number of concepts, fears, memories, and various emotions. Often we associate specific foods with particular times or emotional states from our past. In order to see our foods and ourselves for what they and we really are, these "added on" realities need to be allowed to dissolve.

This leads us to make certain reorientations in the way we see our lives, our goals, our habits, and ourselves. In psychological terms, this process is often called *cognitive restructuring*, which simply means "changing our mind." For people who chronically overeat, a fundamental part of this process involves discovering what negative thought patterns lead us to overeat. Often these patterns are habitual, and can be replaced with more positively directed images. In many cases, chronic negative thought patterns are related to certain situations in our lives, having to do with our occupation, family relationships, or friendships, or with personal goals we consistently fail to meet. An example of positive reorientation would be to examine our larger goals and organize them into stages, consciously setting smaller "sub-goals" that we can more realistically attain in a shorter time. At the same time, we can begin to regularly put ourselves in contact with people, ideas, or other things we find inspire us, and practice cultivating the image of patience.

One of the classic features of such thought-habit restructuring is to identify when we are feeling frustrations, irritations, anxieties, or other feelings that may lead to overeating or to a tightening of our bodies, and teach ourselves to channel this energy into some type of positive, creative action. For many beginning macrobiotics, simply learning about all the different foods and cooking techniques occupies a fair amount of time. However, while it is tempting to use food itself as our prime creative outlet, this can lead to problems. For many overweight people, focusing too much on diet, even when it is proper diet, can eventually lend itself to compulsive patterns or obsessive thinking. While we cannot let ourselves forget the intrinsic importance of food, putting *too much* focus on food can lead us to become one-sided.

We have to remember that when we are truly healthy, we naturally "eat to live." An obsession with food, regardless of its quality, can result in our "living to eat." In the long run, recovery from eating disorders requires that we learn to find a sense of fulfillment in our daily lives, whether it be through our work, through art, or through some other form of creative contribution to the world.

The Commonsense Perspective on View of Life ⎯⎯⎯

While this area largely overlaps with the above discussion of thinking and behavior, a few points bear restatement here. In any form of eating disorder, the act of eating is often being used to fill a void which needs to be filled by other aspects of life. Though we might not have realized it consciously before learning about macrobiotics, we all know that our food is creating us. When our self-image, sense of self-worth and self-respect, or sense of the direction of our lives is unclear, it is only natural that we look to our food to provide that clarity.

And when we are following an eating pattern that maintains our harmony with nature, our food *does* help to provide that sense of clarity. It is a common experience for people who begin eating macrobiotically, sheerly with the intention of relieving a physical health problem, to find their lives gaining increased clarity on many levels.

Nonetheless, it would be a mistake to use the fact that we are eating properly as a way to avoid taking responsibility for our lives. Food cannot fulfill a void left by an unfulfilled career direction, a lack of friends, or a habitual unwillingness to express ourselves. To help keep food in its proper perspective, several thoughts may be kept in mind:

- *Food is creating me.* Therefore, I would do well to choose my food with care and foresight, and treat it with respect as I prepare and consume it.

- *Food is a gift from nature.* Understanding and remembering this fact automatically strengthens my sense of gratitude, whenever I prepare or eat food.

- *Food is giving me life.* This gift is priceless, and it is being given to me to share and redistribute. How would I most enjoy passing this gift on to others? Now that nature and food have created me, what shall I create?

---

1 *Diabetes and Hypoglycemia*, p. 43.
2 *East West Journal*, August 1985, p. 60.
3 *Time*, March 14, 1983, p. 75.
4 *Fit or Fat*, Covert Bailey, p. 6 ff.
5 Bailey, p. 8.
6 Bailey, pp. 8 & 11.
7 *Eating Disorders*, Hilde Bruch, MD, p. 6.
8 "The Roots of Gluttony," Konner, Melvin, *Science Digest*, September, 1982.
9 Bruch, p. 29.
10 *Human Nutrition and Dietetics*, Davidson et al., Churchill Livingstone, London 1979, p. 246.
11 *Lancet*, March 12, 1977.
12 *Emotional Aspects of Obesity*, W.W. Hamburger, Med. Clin. N. Amer., Ref. in Bruch, p. 123.
13 Bruch, p. 127.
14 "Society Abhors Obesity," *Hartford Courant*, Hartford, Connecticut, February 23, 1985.
15 Cf. *Diabetes and Hypoglycemia*, pp. 57–58.
16 The "ob/ob strain" of mice and the "Zucker strain" of rats; *Human Nutrition and Dietetics*, op. cit.
17 *East West Journal*, p. 42.
18 Bruch, p. 26–28.
19 "The Roots of Gluttony," op. cit.
20 "Dieting: The Losing Game," op. cit.
21 "Topics in Primary Care Medicine: Approach to Obese Patients," Eugene V. Boisaubin, MD, *The Western Journal of Medicine*, May 1984, p. 794.
22 "Mechanisms for the Control of Body-Weight," Payne and Dugdale, *Lancet*, March 12, 1977, p. 583.
23 A 1970 study of New York City residents showed these varying rates of incidence of obesity: upper class: 5 percent, middle class: 17 percent, and lower class: 30 percent. From *Human Nutrition and Dietetics*, op. cit., p. 245.
24 "The New American Diet," *Solstice*, Vol. I, No. 1, p. 13, Macrobiotic Association of Rochester, Rochester NY.
25 Trowell, p. 21.
26 *Diet and Nutrition*, Rudolph Ballentine, MD, pp. 500, 503.
27 "The Fat Child," *Parents*, Vol. S8 (11): 111, 1983.
28 For discussion of this subject, please refer to the authors' *Allergies*.

5. Understanding Overweight ━━━━

To understand how illness develops, we can compare the human form to that of a tree. A tree absorbs its nourishment through its roots, transforming the elements from its food—the soil—into sap. That sap is circulated up into the trunk, branches, leaves, and finally to the fruit and flowers. If the quality of the soil is too acid, or too alkaline, or in some other way imbalanced, or if the tree's root system is impaired, the leaves and fruits can't develop normally, and they eventually deteriorate.

In human beings, it is the balance and quality of our food (our "soil") and the condition of our intestinal "roots," particularly the intestinal villi, that is transformed into our bloodstream, determining the health or sickness, balance or imbalance, of our cells, tissues, and organs.

In the human body, the nervous system and brain are analogous to the tree's fruits. The crown of our physical development, they are supported by our trunk and branches, our skeletal and muscular systems. If our nourishment is not balanced properly, the body—including the circulatory organs, liver, kidneys, and endocrine glands—work hard to correct the imbalance and absorb any toxins, to protect the fragile brain. Out of the need to keep our bloodstream properly balanced, in terms of its temperature, alkalinity, glucose level, and various other balances, our body makes every effort to neutralize and discharge the toxins produced by normal metabolism.

By the time obvious symptoms of ill health begin to appear, the body has already been grappling with an unhealthy inner condition, often for quite a long time, striving to maintain balance. Overweight generally begins as a part of this effort. This is best understood by examining the progressive stages of this process.

The Progressive Development of Illness ━━━━

1. Normal Discharge. In a normal state of health, elimination of wastes occurs through the processes of urination, bowel movement, respiration (exhaling carbon dioxide together with other wastes), perspiration, and the caloric and energetic discharge of physical and mental activity. Menstruation, childbirth, and lactation provide women with additional means of cleansing themselves, often allowing them to adjust more smoothly to their environment and live slightly longer than men. Historically, men have compensated for this lack with additional vigorous activity.

For most people these daily mechanisms are not quite enough to keep the body completely clean of accumulated wastes; periodically, we often effect a bodywide "housecleaning" by raising the level of our discharging, such as through an annual "cold" or fever. Additional examples of such mildly *abnormal discharge* would include diarrhea, coughing and sneezing, mild infections (such as middle ear or throat infections), and temporarily elevated behavior, such as anger outburts or hysterical laughing.

In cases where even periodic abnormal discharge is insufficient to balance our internal condition, our system gears itself up to levels of *chronic and extreme discharge*. Extreme discharge would include severe menstrual cramps, skin disease, persistent high fevers, and periodic wild or extreme outbursts of behavior and thinking. Chronic discharge includes "nervous" behaviorial habits and distinctive mannerisms, allergies, chronic menstrual discomforts, chronic bowel troubles, chronic infections, and others. At this point, since our means of discharging are no longer keeping pace with the buildup of toxins and imbalances from our daily food intake, we are already beginning the next stage of illness.

2. Accumulation and Storage. As our ability to eliminate waste is exhausted, the body employs a different means of self-protection, and begins to accumulate excess as stores of fat, mucus, and water, together with various excess minerals and different waste compounds. Storage itself is a natural process which occurs during normal health; the body stores glucose in the form of glycogen, stores amino acids in the liver and muscle tissue, and creates stores of usable fat throughout the body. However, at this stage of illness, this process is elevated to *abnormal* levels. Fat begins to accumulate in the muscle tissue (like "well-marbleized" meats), including the fine muscular walls of the various body organs. A layer of oils, fats, and mucus often accumulates just under the skin and along the lining of the intestines, beginning to block both the eliminating function of the pores and the processes of intestinal absorption and elimination. This further decreases our discharging ability and interferes with our nutritional balance, which leads to still further accumulation of wastes.

Wastes also begin to accumulate toward all the body's natural discharge pathways. These include not only the skin and intestines, but also the sinuses, nasal passages and bronchia, the kidneys and bladder, reproductive organs, the breasts, and throat. This process forms the foundation of more serious diseases, such as gallstones, tumors, and organ degeneration. For example, though modern medicine says that benign breast lumps and uterine fibroid tumors are not related to malignancies (that is, having the one does not mean the other will develop), we can see that *benign* lumps and tumors are a serious indication that we are reaching the limits of our capacity to store toxic excesses, and a process such as cancer may soon be following. This is why we often term extreme chronic discharges and well-progressed benign accumulations as "pre-cancer."[1]

Just as we express the process of discharge on mental as well as physical levels, the various levels of accumulation also occur on mental, emotional, and psychological levels. During this stage we begin to supress feelings and reactions, and to build up excessive stores of various imbalanced thoughts and emotions. While we are beginning the formation of cholesterol and mucus deposits, stones, cysts, and other physical stores, this process is paralleled by the formation of imbalanced attitudes, concepts, complexes, and emotional disturbances. As the physical image of our body grows distorted, so does our image of ourselves, and of life in general.

At the level of *extreme accumulation*, we begin to enter the next stage of illness.

3. *Extreme Storage and Degeneration.* At the extreme point of accumulation, our body eventually begins to adapt to our imbalanced internal environment by changing structurally. This is the process we call "degenerative disease." Depending upon the quality and location of our particular forms of excess, this can take many different forms. If towards the pancreas, we may develop diabetes; if towards the joints, arthritis; towards the liver, cirrhosis; and towards the heart or cardiac arteries, various forms of cardiovascular disease. Cancer is another example of this process. At this stage, we have exhausted our body's capacity to adapt to our everyday habits of food and drink and still maintain normal human form and function. Thus, degenerative illnesses could be called *extreme adaptation*, but the adaptation is so extreme that it endangers our very life.

Mentally and emotionally, our sense of self begins to break down or be radically altered. The framework of thoughts and concepts that comprise our view of life cannot maintain itself without some extreme form of distortion. This was described at the end of Chapter 2.

The key issue to understand here is that in the early stages of illness, we are not "sick" in the usual sense of the term. People often react, for example, to an annual "common cold" or periodic fever, by saying, "Oh, my immune system must be weak." Actually, such *sickness of adjustment* is a sign that the immune system is functioning properly. These mild adjustments are acting to protect our organism from more serious accumulations, and to keep the body clean. It is when such discharges become extreme or chronic in nature that we should realize that we are creating long-term imbalances, and begin to reflect carefully on the way in which we are living.

As we will see, the symptom of overweight can occur at any one of these stages. But before we see how this progression relates to weight problems, let us look at the problem of overweight in terms of yin and yang.

Is Overweight Yin or Yang?

Using what we have learned about yin and yang, it is not hard to see that overweight itself is generally a more yin condition. Physically speaking, fat itself is more yin as compared with carbohydrate or protein; this is why fat or oil have a greater capacity to hold heat (yang). In fact, this is one of fat's values to the body; because it is more yin, it can hold more calories.

Looking at the way fat storage and glucose storage work in the body gives us a more detailed view. Glucose is often stored in the liver and muscle tissue as glycogen, which is also called "animal starch" because it is the form of carbohydrate animals create. The conversion of glucose to glycogen occurs by the subtraction of one molecule of water (yin), making glycogen more yang and less easily dissolved.[2] When glycogen is stored in a body cell, it can take up a maximum of 15 percent of the cell's volume; the rest is used for water and various other cell elements. This is a ratio we often find occurring in nature—one part yang with seven parts yin.[3] Glycogen is more yang, while the rest of the cell is more yin. In the cellular storage of *fat*, this ratio is reversed: a fat cell may be composed of 85 percent actual fat, with only 15 percent remaining space for other cell elements. In a fat cell, in other words, the same 1:7 ratio is represented, but with fat being yin, and the rest of the cell being yang.

Fig. 9 Maximum Cellular Storage Space for Glycogen and Fat

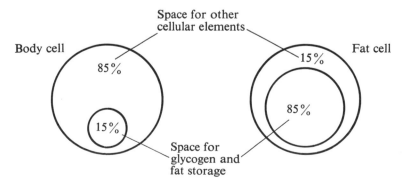

Another way to see that fat is very yin is the fact that fat will rise to the top of water and float. This is why we can determine the Lean Body Mass by accurate measurement of how a person floats in a water tank.

Overweight itself is a condition of expansion—the body grows larger. Overeating is itself also more yin: eating a greater volume is more yin, and makes us more yin, as compared with eating a smaller volume of the same food.

We have seen a variety of more yin symptoms that often accompany overweight, including a greater tendency towards inactivity and a tendency for the symptoms of diabetes. Statistically, women are more prone to obesity than are men; women are naturally more yin, while men are physically more yang. Further, recent studies have revealed two overweight body types, those that tend toward weight gain in the upper body, sometimes called "Apples," and those that tend more toward weight gain in the lower body, called "Pears." Since yang excess tends to settle lower in the body, and yin excess higher in the body, we can classify "Apples" as relatively more yin, and "Pears" as relatively more yang. If overweight is more yin in general, we would expect that overweight "Apples" are more at risk for accompanied health problems than overweight "Pears." This is exactly what research has found.[4]

Fig. 10   Yin and Yang Distribution of Body Fat

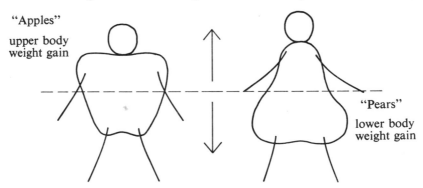

"Apples"

upper body
weight gain

"Pears"

lower body
weight gain

From these observations, we might conclude that overweight is a more yin condition, caused by the overconsumption of excessively yin food and drink, including refined foods, sugar, oil and fat, alcohol, and dairy products. And in fact, this is often the case: many people find it quite easy to lose substantial amounts of excess weight by eliminating these items from their diets. However, it would be a mistake to be satisfied with this simple conclusion. In reality, the situation is usually a bit more involved.

The Dynamics of Overweight

Two fundamental principles of yin and yang are, "Everything has a front and a back," and, "The greater the front, the greater the back."[5] This simply means that every coin has two sides; the side we see is the "front," while the side we don't see, the "back," generally has an opposite nature.

As an example, people who are very mild-mannered on the surface often have a strong resolve or stubborn streak, which they don't easily show. Conversely, a person with a very overbearing or domineering "front" usually hides a deep sense of insecurity or vulnerability. Following the second of the principles stated above, we can guess that the tougher a person acts, the greater will be his "soft spot."

As a more physical example, we can see that water retention is generally caused by fluids, watery foods, and sugar (the metabolism of simple sugar produces a large amount of water). But, what causes this excessive water to accumulate, for example, in the ankles, breast, or face? Often it is the excessive consumption of salt or sodium-rich animal foods (yang), that attracts the excess fluid and holds it in a particular area. In this example, fluid is the "front," salt the "back." And simply reducing fluid or sugar intake does not always solve the problem; often we must find some way to eliminate the excessive salt first.

The same precise principle often applies to overweight. The overweight condition is the "front," which in this case is yin. There is usually a "back," which is more yang. The greater the overweight, the greater the hidden yang factors are liable to be. And as in the case of water retention, it is often difficult to permanently eliminate the excess weight without at the same time dissolving or eliminating those yang factors.

Normally, we balance mildly yin and mildly yang factors together, maintaining a dynamic state of balance. This is analogous to two people of different natures existing together in a dynamic balance, which we would call "love." In cases of overweight, there are usually more extreme factors of both yin *and* yang existing together in a delicate balance which can escalate towards a dangerous level. This would be more analogous to the state of tension that leads to *war*.

This is one reason simple weight-reduction diets don't work. By simply eliminating the front, the yin excess, overweight can be temporarily changed. But the overweight itself may have been maintaining a form of balance with more yang factors, and if these underlying factors are not dealt with, the attraction to gain back weight will be stronger than ever.

This is similar to the pattern of alcoholism, compulsive eating of sweets, and drug addictions. In all these examples, the obvious symptoms are an irresistible attraction to dangerously high consumption of extremely yin substances. But these compulsions are very difficult to change, unless we find the underlying extremely yang factors that are fueling them and change those as well.

Let's explore what some of these underlying yang factors might be.

Common Yang Factors in Overweight ─────────

1. *Extreme Yang Factors in Diet.* The most direct factor is extremely yang foods in our diet. These include: meat and eggs; aged, salty cheeses; poultry and more active fish (red-meat and blue-skinned fish), and especially, salted and smoked fish; excessive salt in general, especially commercial refined salt; and the lack of good quality, mildly yin foods, especially lightly cooked vegetables.

   It should be remembered that such foods can build up in the body and remain as stored accumulations for long periods. Even though we may avoid eating any meat or cheese at all for several months, the substance and the effects of these foods may still be present.

2. *Yang Constitutional Factors.* Everybody has a uniquely different set of constitutional features, depending upon our parents' and ancestors' physical constitution, our parents' way of eating during the period lasting from our conception until we were weaned, and to some extent by our own dietary patterns in childhood.

   A more yin constitution is characterized by such features as a more elongated or delicate bone structure, a thinner and more vertically oriented face, sloping shoulders and a more slight appearance, more narrow palms and longer, thinner fingers; and a more quiet, romantic, intellectual, or passive personality type. In some cases, longer arms and legs and a taller overall height can also signify a more yin constitution.

   Signs of a more yang constitution include a sturdier frame with thicker, more heavy-set bones, a more square or broad face, broader shoulders and a stockier appearance, thicker or more square palms with shorter, thicker fingers; and a more active, practical, boisterous or outgoing personality type. Short stature also signifies a more compact, yang structure, though a person may be relatively tall and still be judged as more yang according to the other features listed above.

   Neither yin nor yang is considered to be "preferable," nor does either imply the person will experience greater or poorer health. They are simply different areas of emphasis in the range of human individuality. However, one's constitutional type does have implications in our daily diet. The chronic overconsumption of strong yin will usually cause a greater immediate imbalance, and a more rapid deterioration, in a person with a more yin constitution. Conversely, someone with a very yang constitution has less tolerance for extremely yang foods. This is explained by the principle that, while opposites attract one another, similar poles tend to repel each other. A person who is already quite yang, by virtue of his constitution, cannot easily absorb much excess yang from his daily diet, but will naturally be attracted to larger volumes of more yin food and drink.

This is not to say that having a certain constitutional type "causes" a certain health condition. Nothing could be further from the truth: it is possible for someone of any constitutional character to enjoy good health. *But for a person who is already quite yang by constitution, the effects of extremely yang foods will be further exaggerated.* This person's attraction to extreme yin will grow proportionately, as will the resulting tendency to create an extremely yin condition such as obesity. Among people who are extremely obese, it is rare to find one with a distinctly yin constitution. One cannot significantly alter or change one's constitution, nor would it necessarily be desirable to do so even if it were possible. *But we can change what we eat every day*, so that it balances our constitution rather than fights it.

Eating meat, eggs, and salty cheeses is not the only example of this. If our constitution is emphatically more yang, it is possible even within the scope of macrobiotics to eat a diet that is uncomfortably yang. Suppose an individual is using slightly stronger amounts of natural sea salt and salt-based seasonings, cooking foods consistently for a longer period, regularly using those grains and vegetables which are slightly more yang, eating more than an occasional serving of fish, and seldom eating any natural desserts or salads. This would, strictly speaking, seem to qualify as "macrobiotic." And it would indeed be an appropriate way to eat for some people, at certain times, to help balance a more yin condition.

This general approach to eating will usually have the effect of making an overweight person slightly more yang, that is, losing weight by discharging excess yin, such as water and fat. At first, an individual will gain more energy, feel clearer, and generally experience an increasing sense of well being. Over time, though, as he contracts further, he may begin to feel uncomfortable, and even lose energy. At this point, he is beginning to feel the fact that this diet is slightly too yang for him: his *condition* has changed, and now his intrinsically more yang nature requires a shift towards a more moderately yin pattern of eating. If this is not understood, it is easy

84

to be eventually overwhelmed by an attraction to stronger forms of yin, leading into the familiar cycle of extreme yin foods and recurring weight gain.

3. *Yang Environmental and Lifestyle Factors.* Finally, aspects of our everyday life and the world around us can cause one to feel more yang, aggravating the imbalances described above. The most commonly experienced yang factor from everyday life is *pressure*—all types of pressure. One of the strongest pressures felt by the overweight is society's attitudes towards weight. These values are expressed in commercial advertising and fashion magazines, for example, which create a tremendous pressure to be as slim as possible. A full day of looking at fashion-model advertisements and hearing criticisms of fatness can create enough sensation of pressure to produce the very real desire for strong yin, such as eating a bag of cookies.

It is important to understand where this pressure originates. In traditional societies, even though overweight occurred far less than in modern societies, it was also looked down upon much less. In our modern society, tolerance for overweight has *decreased* as our overweight condition itself has *increased*. This is another example of the principle that similarities tend to repel each other. A person who looks down upon us and considers that we are ugly or unattractive because we are overweight, is doing so because he himself is also out of balance. When someone with a naturally healthy condition encounters an overweight person, his natural reaction is to see the excess weight simply for what it is. It does not interfere with the normal enjoyment of the other person's company any more than would the knowledge that the person had diabetes or an ulcer. Though there may be little one can do to change society's attitudes overnight, it is possible to gain a better understanding of such pressures, and so be less susceptible to their extreme effects.

Another example of environmental and lifestyle pressure is an extremely fast-paced, hectic, or over-mechanized environment, such as we often experience in our modern cities. This may need to be balanced by regular time in the countryside, or by a compensating environment in the home. Extraordinarily high self-expectations and overly harsh self-imposed goals can be another form of pressure. Likewise, a strong emotional confrontation, shock, or other form of "trauma" can create an overly yang, contracting feeling. For people with an already overly yang condition created by daily food, and particularly when accompanied with an already more yang constitution, such circumstances can be the yang "trigger" that results in the response of active weight gain.

While we cannot control others' actions, we can control our own reaction to them. By gaining a deeper understanding of our circumstances and others' behavior, and by exercising judgement in creating our home environment to balance our everyday lives, we can learn to neutralize the extreme effects of such factors.

The True Origin and Causes of Overweight

Overweight has two general causes. First, it originates with the loss of natural contact with nature and the environment. This occurs on two basic levels. Externally, our skin loses its ability to eliminate and breathe, cutting us off from our surroundings. Living in an increasingly artificialized environment, including the use of synthetic fabrics worn next to the skin, living most of our lives within concrete enclosures with little fresh air circulation, constant exposure to fluorescent lighting, and other similar factors, contributes to our increasing separation from the natural world around us.

Internally, the surface of our digestive organs becomes congested and compacted with fat and mucus, reducing the exchange between our food and our bloodstream through absorption. Though this separation is hidden from view, it is even more critically important to our harmony with nature than the external, more visible factors. This is the point where our environment actually becomes us.

This separation, as we saw in previous chapters, stems from the loss of our traditional way of eating. Our modern artificial, scientific, and commercialized dietary pattern separates us from nature both in its immediate physical effects and, in the long run, on mental and psychological levels as well.

The second cause of overweight lies in the extremes of yin and yang in our lives, and most particularly in our diet. Because we are losing our natural connection with nature, we grow unable to correct these imbalances through intuitive adjustment in our diet and lifesytle. Increasingly inflexible and extreme of mind, we react to the extremes in our body and life in extreme ways, and the cycle escalates.

The Progressive Development of Overweight and Obesity

Overweight develops in three stages, which we can call early, middle, and late; these could also be termed the adaptive stage, maladaptive stage, and degenerative stage.

During the *adaptive* first stage, we consume an excess of yin food and drink, often in an effort to balance a more tightened, yang inner condition or external circumstance, or both. Initially, this excess yin may be discharged through diarrhea, chronic infections, or other means, but at some point it begins to accumulate. Being yin, it tends to move to the periphery, where it takes the form of excess body fat and water. While this is not a healthy way of maintaining balance, this stage is essentially a *protective* process, through which the person may be avoiding a more serious condition.

Often, during this stage, the same process is happening on an emotional and psychological level. Though more yang feelings of anger, aggression, and self-justification may be gathering internally, these may be balanced by an increasing posture of defensiveness. Frequently more yin emotions, such as depression, lack of confidence, and the sense of being victimized, develop as a counterpart to the yin physical condition. This corresponds to what is sometimes called the "active" phase of weight gain. While still in this stage, overweight conditions can usually be changed quite easily, and in a fairly short period of time.

The second, or *maladaptive* stage occurs as our metabolism gradually adjusts itself to our overweight condition. This is similar to what is sometimes called the "stationary" or "stable" phase, when our body settles into the pattern of being overweight and is less easily moved out of it by simple reducing methods. The so-called "active" phase is more yang, while this "stationary" phase is more yin. In other words, during this second phase, the yin, overweight condition begins to permeate our whole system; our actual weight may no longer be increasing, but we are gradually becoming more yin in other ways.

Another way of seeing this is to realize that the first phase is more a change in *quantity*, that is, our own physical bulk is increasing. This second phase represents a more *qualitative* change, and can occur in many ways. In terms of our endocrine system, we may now begin to develop towards diabetes, thyroid problems, or reproductive-hormone changes. In our circulatory system we may find our blood pressure and cholesterol levels increasing; our skeletal and *articular* (joint) systems may begin to develop towards various forms of arthritis or *osteoporosis* (bone calcium loss).

At the same time, our perception of ourselves and the world is profoundly altered. Extreme feelings or attitudes become ingrained and habitual, and we resist change far more stubbornly than during the early stage. We are no longer truly adapting to the world around us, but are rather beginning to adapt to an extreme world we have created inside ourselves, both physically and mentally. Recovering from overweight at this stage will require more extensive reorientation to reestablish a healthy balance.

In the late or *degenerative* stage, overweight becomes a life-threatening issue. It is not that the weight itself endangers us so directly, but the associated maladaptations now progress to the point of full-blown degenerative syndromes, such as cancer, heart disease, or severe diabetes. Our way of balancing the extremes within us has reached the limits of human tolerance.

At this point, we can say that we have in some way lost contact with nature, and with reality—or to put it differently, the *new* reality we have created within ourselves has become firmly entrenched. Because this created reality is so at odds with the harmony of nature that created us, this situation is highly unstable. Even when it does not put our life in immediate danger, it can so interfere with the quality of life as to make our existence one of constant misery. People do not generally die, for example, of arthritis, and Type II diabetes is often somewhat controlled with oral drugs, as is hypertension. Though our lifespan is shortened, we continue to survive. But it becomes almost impossible to really enjoy our everyday lives as free human beings.

One cannot necessarily judge at which of these three stages a person is at the moment, sheerly on the basis of size or fat percentage. A person of an extremely strong, yang constitution may gain a tremendous amount of weight while still in the first stage, and maintain himself at that stage for many years without any substantial development of degenerative disease. On the other hand, a person who is only fifteen or twenty pounds overweight may have developed some deeply ingrained overweight emotional patterns and serious illnesses.

Probably the most accurate measure of how far progressed a person's condition has become—aside from obvious information such as the actual appearance of serious diseases—is the ease, flexibility, and speed with which the person can adapt, change himself, and recover.

The Macrobiotic Approach to Recovery from Overweight

In many cases, simply changing to a macrobiotic way of eating alone will recover normal weight and physical health. In other cases, additional physical means can help, and changing one's overall perspective is necessary to make these changes deep and lasting ones. In some cases, those changes that do *not* directly involve diet can be so important that dietary change itself is not effective or not possible until other changes have occurred. Dietary change is the fundamental means for recovery. However, generally speaking, the more progressed the condition and the more deeply ingrained the overweight metabolic, emotional, and psychological habits, the more crucial are those changes other than diet.

Below are listed seven general aspects of the macrobiotic approach to recovering from overweight problems.

1. *Dietary Change.* In many cases, simply following the standard macrobiotic approach to eating will result in normalizing weight. This is detailed in Chapter 7.

2. *Specific Dietary Adjustments.* It is often helpful to include specific guidelines and even include specific dishes for a variety of special purposes. For example, certain preparations can help to cleanse the intestines of accumulated mucus and fat deposits; strengthen the kidneys and eliminatory functions; or help dissolve and eliminate deposits of animal fat, animal protein, and salt. It is preferable to follow specific guidelines together with the guidance of an experienced macrobiotic teacher. Some general suggestions are outlined in Chapter 7.

3. *External Treatments.* In cases where the internal organs are heavily congested or have difficulty recovering full function, there are mild, traditional external applications and compresses that can help encourage more rapid change. Again, these are outlined in Chapter 7.

4. *Activity and Body Awareness.* In cases of deep-rooted overweight problems, there is often a distortion of body sense and general lack of awareness of the body. Both to improve circulation, metabolism, and electromagnetic energy flow, and to increase our direct sense of our own body, various types of exercise and activity are extremely helpful.

5. *Lifestyle and Personal Environment.* In order to modify extremes of yin and yang in our lives and to learn to achieve a more balanced life, it is necessary to identify and examine factors in our everyday lifestyle that contribute to extreme feelings, or that serve to cut us off from nature or make us feel isolated. Our personal environment can be modified to help provide more of a sense of natural balance. Occasionally, it may even be necessary to alter our work patterns or change our living place or occupation, if these are contributing in an extreme way to our sense of imbalance.

6. *Emotional and Psychological Self-Reflection.* Since our physical body is a reflection of the image we have of ourselves, it is necessary

for us to be completely honest in evaluating what kind of character and personal traits we see in ourselves, and to explore the ways in which we habitually deal with circumstances and other people. In this process of self-reflection, it is best to avoid complex thinking and elaborate evaluation. We can arrive at a simple, direct, and practical view of what kind of behavior and expression we would like to create, based upon a honest assessment of our basic strengths and weaknesses, and begin to follow a realistic, step-by-step course to realize that vision.

In cases where a serious medical condition exists, it is advisable to make positive lifestyle changes together with the guidance of an appropriate medical professional, preferably one who is in sympathy with natural approaches to health. Likewise, if a serious psychological problem exists, it may be advisable to work together with an experienced psychologist or other counselor. However, it is best not to dwell on our psychological or emotional imbalances more than is necessary to begin moving toward a simpler, more balanced and positive approach to life.

It is also important to remember that seemingly complex psychological and emotional problems are frequently maintained by a chaotic diet. Commonly, such problems grow simpler and easier to dissolve after a short period of following a more balanced diet and recovering a more natural state of health. This can greatly reduce the amount of special counseling or other help that might otherwise be necessary.

7. *View of Life.* This issue is discussed extensively in Chapter 2, and again in Chapter 8. Briefly, the entire effort to reorient our health should be based upon a positive view of life, including an appreciation of the miracle of life and the gift of our own individual lives, and an appreciation of the orderliness of nature and our place within it.

---

[1] This is not the same meaning as the medical term "pre-cancerous," which generally means that some abnormal tissue behavior has already been observed.
[2] *Diabetes and Hypoglycemia*, p. 26 ff.
[3] For example, as we saw before, we have four "canine" teeth as opposed to twenty-eight "vegetarian" teeth. For other examples, please see *The Book of Macrobiotics*.
[4] "Dieting: The Losing Game," *Time*, January 20, 1986.
[5] For a summary of the basic principles of yin and yang, please refer to *The Book of Macrobiotics*.

6. Anorexia Nervosa and Bulimia ▬

> In the month of July she fell into a total supression of her Monthly
> Courses from a multitude of Cares and Passions of her Mind . . . From
> which time her Appetite began to abate, and her Digestion to be bad . . .
> I do not remember that I did ever in all my practice see one, that was
> conversant with the Living so much wasted with the greatest degree of
> a Consumption (like a Skeleton only clad with Skin) yet there was no
> Fever, but on the contrary a coldness of the whole Body . . .[1]

The eighteen year old daughter of one Mr. Duke thus fell ill, from what
the author described as "A Nervous Consumption" in what is generally
credited as the first clinical description of this rare condition. Like generations of anorectic women to follow, she rejected all medications, and
died three months afterward.[2]

Two centuries later another Londoner, Sir William Gull, published
reports of many such cases of self-inflicted starvation accompanied by
what he termed a "morbid mental state." Gull observed that this condition seemed to appear mostly in young women, and coined the term
Anorexia Nervosa, which literally means "lack of appetite stemming
from mental [not physical] causes."[3] At about the same time a French
researcher, Lasegue, reported on eight patients, most of them women
from the ages of fifteen to twenty years, who suffered from a condition
he termed *anoreixie hysterique*, the term which is still used today in
France and Italy.

Though exceedingly rare, the condition of anorexia nervosa or anorexie
hysterique became established as a clinical observation from that time
on. As with obesity, theories on its cause fluctuated with the tides of
scientific advance. Originally considered as a disorder of an exclusively
psychological origin (most likely inherited), anorexia nervosa underwent
the same kind of redefinition as many other conditions during the "endocrine revolution" in the early 1900s. Triggered by a 1914 report by
a physiologist named Simmonds, of a rare pituitary condition accompanied by emaciation (now called *Simmonds disease*), a great number of
theorists began to consider anorexia as an endocrine gland disorder.[4]
Starting in the 1930s the tide began to swing the other way, and anorexia
is now largely considered as a disorder of psychological origins.

Though the condition was known since the late 1800s, it was not until
a century later that it burst upon the public consciousness. All observers

agree that the condition has significantly escalated since about 1970, and dramatically so since 1977. The average age of onset today is about the same as Mr. Duke's daughter's eighteen years; this means that the recent dramatic increase has centered on the generation of women born after 1960.

It is estimated that one in every 250 adolescent girls suffers from anorexia. A college survey (cited in Chapter 1) found that from 25 percent to 33 percent of college-age women are involved in some type of eating disorder. While the disorder has been known to afflict people of all economic backgrounds and most age groups, the vast majority still fit the profile observed by Gull, Lasegue, and Morton: 97 percent are white, mostly from middle and upper income brackets in affluent countries (particularly North America, Western Europe, and Australia), most experience onset of the condition between the ages of eleven and twenty-two, and nearly all are women.

In addition, the typical anorectic is highly intelligent and articulate, often appearing unusually outgoing, cheerful, and competent. She is rarely perceived as being a "problem child" until the onset of the eating disorder; less than 15 percent are observed to have had any prior problems with overweight. Though anorexia is often popularly associated with being an only child, one authority notes that 80 percent are actually second or third children. In fact, the consistent "normalcy" of personal and health profiles of many anorectics only emphasizes the mystery of how such an extreme pattern of behavior could develop.

The profile for bulimia is not essentially different, but for several factors. For example, more men (from 10 percent to 15 percent, according to one estimate[5]) suffer from bulima. The clinical picture varies more broadly, and there is not the history of clinical definition that we can trace with anorexia.

Strictly speaking, bulimia is not a single condition, but a general description of a range of eating disorders that overlap to a greater or lesser extent with anorexia nervosa. The term itself means a voracious appetite—literally, "the hunger of an ox."[6] Bulimia is most commonly associated with the practice of periodic "bingeing and purging"; in this pattern, a typical bulimic may eat as much as 15,000 calories in a day (perhaps a week's supply or more), and then through self-induced vomiting, disgorge it all in order to keep from gaining any weight. One bulimic's typical "binge" is described below:

2   pounds of vanilla sandwich cookies with vanilla filling
1   pint of vanilla ice milk
1   pint of butter pecan ice cream

2 quarts of skim milk
4 waffles
1 loaf of white bread
½ pound of butter   } for French toast
6 eggs
1 bottle of maple syrup
1 pound of Ritz crackers
½ pound of potato salad
½ pound of bakery cookies, assorted
1 packaged crumb coffee cake (1 pound)
2 ice cream sandwiches
2 yogurts
10 cream-filled chocolate cupcakes[7]

It is not unusual for a bulimic to follow one such binge, after a cycle of vomiting, with another several hours later, and even a third. This pattern may continue for several days at a time. Cases where this cycle alternates with days of severe "intake limiting" (eating perhaps only 300 to 600 calories per day), are sometimes referred to as *Anorexia/Bulimia* or *Bulimarexia*. However, many people practice a cycle of only the bingeing and purging itself, without any anorexic behavior. This last group includes many degrees of such practices, as well as the use of laxatives, diuretics, and emetics. This pattern, which may be much more widespread than previously identified, frequently does not share the same psychological and behaviorial profiles as anorexia and anorexia/bulimia.

The Clinical Profile ────────────────────────────

The physical dangers from these disorders are considerable: in at least 1 out of 8 cases, anorexia nervosa results in death. And aside from mortality, the extremes to which the body is pushed in both anorexia and bulimia can exact a terrifying toll on health.

Below are listed the criteria for clinical diagnosis of anorexia nervosa:

- loss of 20 percent of body weight [the exact inverse of obesity; in many cases, weight drops considerably lower]
- *amenorrhea* (lose of menstrual period) [together with a disturbance of the normal balance of female hormones]
- thinning hair
- *lanugo* (a downy growth of body hair, normally seen only in infants)
- constipation
- dry, flaking skin [and parched lips]

- lowered blood pressure (80/50 is not uncommon)
- lowered body temperature (97° to 95°F is common)
- lowered pulse rate (60 to 39 beats per minute)[8]

Often accompanying these features are: the flat refusal to eat more than a bare minimum, with an obsessive fear of gaining weight; profound perceptual disturbances, such as an exaggerated sensitivity to some stomach sensations or complete lack of awareness of normal stomach contractions; a generally obsessive nature, such as compulsive hyperactivity; an overwhelmingly strong sense of commitment to the anorectic condition; and a number of other pronounced psychological patterns that will be described presently.

The same general constellation of symptoms applies to bulimic sufferers, depending upon the degree to which they practice nutritional deprivation. In addition, the frequent and sometimes violent vomiting of bulimia can lead to three further classic symptoms:

1. Due to the regular presence of the stomach's powerful hydrochloric acid in the mouth, the teeth may be badly impaired.
2. The mechanical action of periodic vomiting can lead to abrasions and bleeding of the esophagus; in some cases this has even resulted in rupture, which can be fatal.
3. The periodic vomiting also leads to a disturbed *electrolyte* (electrically charged minerals) balance, particularly with chronically low levels of potassium and chloride. Since potassium and sodium ions regulate the exchange of the body's nerve impulses, this can prevent normal neuro-muscular exchanges, leading to *cardiac arrhythmia* (irregular heartbeat) and even heart damage.[9]

Medically speaking, the only therapy for anorexia nervosa other than psychiatric therapy is hospitalization for emergency treatment. Such treatment, which may include direct feeding through a catheter and intravenous supplementation of vital nutrients, is generally applied only when the patient's life is threatened by severe emaciation. Otherwise, the current approaches to anorexia are exclusively psychiatric, and admittedly, the techniques of routine psychiatric therapy are often not effective.[10]

The Psychological Profile

As with obesity, nobody really knows to what degree the physical changes that accompany anorexia may be caused by a psychological condition, or how much the common psychological patterns may be a result of the severe metabolic changes themselves. There have been many attempts to make sense out of the wide range of common psychological features exhibited by anorectics, to try to discern a central theme. Some of these common features include:

- *phobias*, especially concerning body appearance;
- *feelings of inferiority* and *paranoid fears of criticism* from others;
- *drastic perceptual changes* and *denial* of seemingly obvious facts;
- *"splitting,"* the tendency to see things in rigidly absolute terms such as "absolutely good" and "completely bad" with no middle ground or sense of moderation;
- *obsessional thinking* and *obsessive-compulsive rituals*, such as a fanatic preoccupation with the precise details of food volumes, meal schedules, and of time and schedules in general;
- *alternating patterns* of outward compliance and geniality alternating with *a hyperconservative rigidity* and even violent temper tantrums;
- and periods of deep *depression* and *anxiety*, alternating with the apparently complete disappearance of these feelings.

Dr. Bruch has differentiated between what she calls *genuine* or *primary* and *atypical* versions of the disorder. While no pattern is apparent in the "atypical" group, she states that the pattern of psychological features of the genuine syndrome is "amazingly uniform."[11] She classifies these features into three general categories, described below.

1. Pronounced delusional misperceptions of the body. It is often not so much that anorectics refuse to acknowledge how thin they are: they often literally *see themselves as larger*. It is common for an anorectic patient to overestimate the dimensions of the hips, buttocks, thighs, waist, and bust by as much as 50 percent.

> Another girl of 19 [upon showing her doctor two pictures of herself, one from earlier when she was normal weight and one of her emaciated self] . . . admitted that she had trouble seeing a difference, though she knew there was one, and that she had been trying to correct this. When she looks at herself in a mirror then she sometimes can see that she is too skinny, 'But I can't hold onto it.' She may remember it for an hour but then begins to feel again that she is much larger.[12]

2. Disturbance in the accuracy of interpreting internal body stimuli. Aside from the misperception of size, anorectics are often completely oblivious to such sensations as measurable stomach contractions, extremes of hot and cold, and fatigue. Consequently, for example, it is common for an anorectic person to drive herself to the very limits of physical activity without sensing that she is physiologically exhausted. On the other hand, ingesting the merest amount of food may immediately trigger the sense of being hugely full.

Awareness of sexual feelings may also disappear, as may the awareness of various emotional states, such as anxiety. For example, when in an emotionally highly charged situation, an anorectic may feel she is perfectly at ease and wonder quite innocently why she has moist palms, a dry mouth, and a flushed face.

3. A paralyzing sense of ineffectiveness. The anorectic's sense of her utter inability to have any effect on the world or events around her, is often undetected by the casual observer. In terms of yin and yang, this is an extremely yin emotional state, and it is often "camouflaged" by compensating extremely yang expressions. The obvious (more yang) patterns of hypercontrol, fanatic rigidity, and stubborn defiance and denial, are desperate attempts to cover up the internal sense of profound hopelessness. This last trait, according to Dr. Bruch, contains the key to effective therapy. "If the therapist communicates his awareness of the patient's sense of helplessness without insult to the patient's fragile self-esteem, meaningful therapeutic involvement becomes possible, avoiding the exhausting power struggle or futile efforts at persuasion that so often characterize treatment of these patients."[13]

One of the difficulties scientists have experienced in gaining a clear understanding of how anorexia develops is the common pattern of "prior normalcy" mentioned earlier. Most patients function so smoothly as children that they are not considered as having problems until they have already reached the point of being severely emaciated.[14] Because there are no widely recognized "early warning signs" of a predisposition to anorexia, existing studies of anorectics are based on direct observations of patients only after the syndrome is in full progress. Any scientific information on what the typical patient may experience *before* the anorexic eating pattern becomes established, is based largely on indirect observations such as parents' recollections, pediatricians' records, and so forth.

Thus, as with obesity, it is difficult for scientists to sort out which symptoms come first, or which may be cause and which may be effect. At the present, there is no course of "prevention" as such, because little is known about the cause, and equally little is known about how to know who is at risk—aside from the obvious course of action of assuming that *all* women under the ages of 18 are at risk. Since the pattern is very difficult to dislodge once it is already established, any sort of early warning signs would be extremely valuable.

The Origins and Causes of Anorexia and Bulimia

In a general sense, these problems are ultimately caused by a similar set of circumstances as that which creates obesity and overweight, though with some special aspects. Again, these circumstances are *a sense of separation from the natural environment*, which in the anorectic patient is drastically severe, and *an extreme imbalance of yin and yang forces* most directly owing to extremes in diet. Let us see how these factors develop to result in anorexia and bulimia.

Separation from the Environment

We have already seen how far an anorectic person is removed from sensing her own body functions, appearance, and even emotional states. This sense of distance from reality is rooted in an extreme congestion and stagnation of fats and mucus, particularly in four areas:

1. *The lining of the intestines,* which is where we come into direct physiological contact with our environment;
2. *Directly underneath the skin,* which has the effect both of dulling sensation and of clogging the pores so that normal elimination and exchange of electromagnetic energies through the skin cannot take place;
3. *In and around the kidneys and adrenal glands,* which serve to regulate our ability to adapt to the environment in general; and
4. *The uterus and reproductive organs,* which we will discuss presently.

The primary causes of this extreme congestion are the overconsumption of extremely fatty foods, particularly *eggs*, *dairy products*, and *meats*, together with refined sugar and foods that produce a chilling effect on the body. These include iced soft drinks, cold orange juice, ice cream or other cold desserts and chilled dairy products, and routine excessive consumption of raw fruits and vegetables, especially those of a tropical or semi-tropical origin, such as tomatoes, eggplants, oranges, figs, and others.

In addition to diet, the childhood home environment often contributes to the anorectic's sense of separation. While certainly not universal, there are a number of recurrent themes that often appear in the parents' relationship with and attitudes toward anorectics during their earlier years (well before the syndrome develops). For example, an anorectic's parents are often described as being "depleted and exhausted ... [resulting in the young pre-anorectic girl's seeing them] as insubstantial and dependent upon the child."[15]

The mother's behavior towards the girl is sometimes referred to as "undifferentiated," that is, with a blurring of the distinction between who is the parent and who the child. The future anorectic's father is often undemonstrative toward the child, and uncomfortable with affection. In such an environment, a young child is encouraged to be independent, and may often feel she needs to supply some of the attributes of leadership, character strength, and emotional resilience that her parents seem unable to provide.

In simple human terms, the child is often not given the chance to really behave as a child. The "insubstantial" and emotionally deficient character of her home life lends life an almost ghostly, unreal sense. Such a background is not in itself enough to create anorexia nervosa. But when coupled with the internal, physiological sense of being "cut off" from the most vital areas of the body, it helps build a tendency towards anorexia.

In cases of bulimia, a similar home pattern may often be present. In addition, there is often a strong emphasis on the modern "consumer ethic." Even when the family is not particularly wealthy, a strong value may be attached to consumption and material goods, with the image that satisfaction in life can most reliably and consistently be gained through material success—the consumption of goods.

Distortion of Yin and Yang

The forces of yin and yang become extremely distorted in cases of eating disorders. This results, again, from dietary extremes. And as in obesity, the underlying condition of rigidity in the digestive tissues tends to make opposite energies sharply polarize as antagonists, rather than come together in balance. An example of this is the anorectic's tendency, noted above, to view everything in highly polarized "black and white" terms, or in the marked alternations of mood. (These, by the way, are often accompanied by extreme swings in blood glucose levels, which are another indicator of yin and yang extremes.)[16]

As an intriguing example of this extreme duality, many anorectics often speak quite openly of feeling like *two* people, a thin one and a fat one. In such cases, the thin "me" is generally seen as the one who gains respect, is highly efficient and productive, but may be secretly selfish;

the fat "me" is seen as more bumbling and incompetent, often looked down upon, clumsy and ineffective, but with a good heart and warm inner personality.[17] Upon examination, we find that these are rather precise caricatures of yin and yang aspects of human nature, the thin representing the yang and the fat being the more yin.

If the preceding chapters were read carefully, readers may have by now understood the crucial difference between the factors that lead to anorexia and those that lead to bulimia. The paragraph above certainly makes it clear. While both are brought about by extremes of both yin and yang, the difference is one of emphasis. Anorexia nervosa is caused more by extreme yin, and bulimia, by extreme yang.

For example, bulimics tend to be more mature, both socially and sexually, and to circulate more in society. That is, their character is more active and yang. Anorectics are generally less adventurous, and tend towards self-seclusion, that is, they are retiring and more yin.

The Yin Nature of Anorexia

One revealing confirmation of the anorexic condition being extremely yin is that anorectics usually perceive themselves as being *big*. Sometimes this feeling of expansion even extends beyond personal boundaries. Dr. Bruch reports on one girl who, on entering the hospital, felt that all the people around her were " ' too large,' and even that the building was too large."[18] While the familiar interpretation of the body as being fat is always seen sheerly as a delusion, *it actually is not a delusion* in the absolute sense. Of course, the anorectic is not "large." But she is *yin*. And in her state of separation from natural energy flow, her sensibilities perceive this imbalance, *accurately*, only misinterpreting it in familiar terms as an imbalance of size.

In order to compensate for their internally yin condition, anorectics attempt to exert an often fanatical control upon themselves and their circumstances, trying in the extreme to be more yang in their behavior. This is most obvious, of course, in their following the most stringent dietary restrictions. By fasting and dietary deprivation, they do indeed make themselves more yang. Unfortunately, this does not result in a healthy balance, but in the escalation of extremes.

The foods that lead to this exaggerated sense of yin are sugar, raw fruits and vegetables and their juices, milk and milk products, and especially combinations of the above, particularly when iced or chilled.

The bulimic, on the other hand, has consumed a great deal of excess yang, usually red meat. It is an irony of language, and perhaps more than that, that we have chosen a term for this condition that translates as

"the hunger of an ox"—for in a literal sense, this is exactly true!
Sensing the extremely tight, yang internal condition, the pre-bulimic
is irresistably moved to expand in some way. Overeating becomes that
way—making herself very yin to unconsciously balance being very yang.
However, she cannot eliminate properly. She is often unable to perspire
due to clogged skin pores. She may be constipated, and even if not,
there is a powerfully entrenched layer of fat and mucus coating the
intestines, which she feels, though is not consciously aware of. Vomiting
becomes the available means of elimination.

Though there are elaborate psychological constructs involved, many
of these are actually created by the person herself, out of the attempt of
her conscious mind to rationally explain what she is doing. To say that
society's pressuring young women to be slim is a cause of bulimia or
anorexia is stretching common sense. Millions of women have experienced this pressure without resorting to extremes of self-starvation, even
to the point of death, or of violent bingeing and purging. While such
environmental factors may play a part, they are more after the fact than
true causes. The true cause stems most directly from a highly imbalanced,
inflexible internal condition, which the young person senses, though
vaguely, and responds to with the natural attempt to balance, albeit in
a destructive way.

Thus far, our explanation leaves two key questions unanswered: why
do these conditions affect predominantly women? And, why is the age
of onset most commonly about the time of puberty or the years immediately thereafter? To understand these problems, we need to understand
something about the nature of male and female sexuality.

The Nature of Human Sexuality

In traditional Chinese medicine there are two body functions, called
triple heater and *heart governor*, which regulate the flow of energy and
temperature between the deepest recesses of the body and the body's
surface. These functions are integrally related to the functions of the
reproductive organs. The energies they regulate are yang and yin, which
we might in this context refer to as "hot" and "cold." For example, in
women who are regularly eating meat, which produces great heat, men-
opause is often accompanied by "hot flashes," which are disturbances
of the triple heater/heart governor balance. On the other hand, a diet of
extreme yin, such as cold drinks and ice cream, can lead someone to
become sexually cold, or frigid.

In anorexia and bulimia, extremes of both heat-producing foods (eggs,
meat, fat) and cold-producing foods (sugar, milk, raw foods, iced drinks,

and chilled foods, etc.) are consumed. But in the anorectic's case, there has been far more emphasis on cooling foods, while the bulimic has consumed relatively more heat-producing foods.

There is an intrinsic difference between male and female sexual organs. Because the male sexual organs are located at the surface of the body, they are subject to more rapid temperature and energy change. Sexually, men tend to "heat up" and "cool down" faster than women. The uterus lies deep within the body, and thus tends to build up a sexual charge far more slowly, and also to dissipate that charge more gradually, than is the case for men. (Not understanding this basic difference, by the way, is one of the most common underlying reasons for sexual miscommunication and unhappiness between sexual partners.)

In the development of these eating disorders, the excessive buildup of fat and "heat" and the freezing effects of chilling foods both profoundly affect the uterus. (They can also affect the prostate or testicles, but not as easily, because these organs lie so near the surface of the body.) This is not so acutely perceived by the body, however, until the onset of menstruation, when the uterus normally begins its natural cycle of discharging and cleansing. When the uterus is unable to do so because of its "frozen" and congested condition, excess begins to build up to intolerable levels in the body, and a state of crisis is precipitated.

In a sense, then, one could say that anorexia and bulimia together comprise a condition of "energetic infertility." In the case of anorexia, the uterus and intestines have become particularly cold, and the image of barrenness eventually pervades the entire person, including her consciousness and behavior. In cases of bulimia, a large amount of "heat" has built up which cannot discharge properly. Sensing this buildup, the person is intuitively afraid to eat for fear of adding to that excess, interpreted by her thoughts as "gaining weight." Since the lower body and skin are unable to fulfill their normal capacity to discharge, excess needs to escape upwards. In some cases, there may be a tendency to perspire just on the face or forehead; the sinuses may continually be clogged and draining; and the person may talk and think very quickly and actively. These are all efforts to discharge energy upwards. Vomiting becomes the answer to this need.

The Macrobiotic Approach to Eating Disorders ———

It is clear that extremes of diet are the prime origin of these conditions, and as with other illnesses, proper diet should be the basis of recovery. However, there are often obvious problems with acting on this principle with anorexia and bulimia. For a bulimic, there may be an overwhelming tendency to be compulsive about food, and it can be difficult at first to practice the diet properly. In cases of anorexia, the person may not be willing to eat macrobiotic food—or *any* food—at all. In both cases, the change in diet *will* change the underlying condition, both physical and psychological, given time. However, it is of course necessary to first come to the point where it is possible to eat this way. Here are several steps that can be taken in that direction.

1. Even before we begin to eat fully macrobiotically, every effort should be made to strongly reduce, and if possible, avoid those particular foods that have created the condition, particularly animal fats, sugar, and cold or cooling foods.

2. The diet itself should be carefully adjusted to compensate for the underlying imbalance. This is an individual matter, and is best pursued together with a competent macrobiotic teacher. In general, an anorectic's diet would be aimed at including more foods to produce warmth in the lower body, which would be more similar to the kind of diet we would normally consume in cooler weather or more northern climates. To help recover from bulimia, a proper diet would tend to include less of such foods, and more foods that produce a relaxing, dissolving, and cooling effect as well as more upward movement. In either case, care should be taken not to consume foods that will tend to congest the intestines, and special dishes can be included that help to dissolve animal fat and strengthen the eliminatory functions.

3. Several types of external treatments can be helpful in accelerating the body's discharge of accumulated excesses and correcting the imbalances discussed above. These treatments will be presented in Chapter 8.

4. The anorectic or bulimic person needs to be helped to see her own body clearly. Clear explanations of what has been going on in the body, including the factors that have led her to be drawn to this pattern, are essential. In some cases (such as the example quoted earlier), even photographs of the person may be helpful to strengthen the image of reality.

5. Together with the above steps, special exercise practices, that can help the person more accurately *feel* her own body, can be very helpful. These would include various types of yoga, tai chi, Do-In self massage, and other traditional forms of martial arts and orderly movement.

6. Continuing the same line of thinking, we can help show the person her own thought patterns. A person suffering from anorexia or

bulimia (and the same would apply to obesity as well) needs to clearly see the elaborate mental constructs she has created to justify and explain the imbalances she feels. These should not only be seen, but also made more simple. Ideally, it is especially helpful to understand these in terms of yin and yang; this helps to remove the social and emotional overtones that have grown around the impulses she feels. If necessary, a competent professional counselor should be consulted regularly until the person has recovered her own sense of natural perspective on what these imbalanced impulses represent.

7. Finally, it is essential to recover a natural sense of the real meaning of food. This would include cultivating a sense of respect and gratitude for food as a manifestation of nature.

---

[1] *Phthisiologia: or a Treatise of Consumption*, Richard Morton, London, 1689.
[2] Quoted from Bruch, p. 211 ff.
[3] "Anorexia Nervosa," Sir Wm. Gull, Trans. Clinii. Soc., London, 7: 22–28, 1874.
[4] In the rest of the book we will refer to anorexia nervosa simply with the term "anorexia"; it should be remembered, however, that the term "anorexia" simply means "having no appetite," and can occur in many contexts other than the syndrome of anorexia nervosa.
[5] Levenkron, p. 65.
[6] From the Greek *bous*, "ox," and *limos*, "hunger or "famine."
[7] Levenkron, p. 77.
[8] Adapted from Levenkron, p. 11.
[9] Levenkron, p. 66.
[10] Levenkron, p. xi.
[11] Bruch, p. 251.
[12] Bruch, p. 90.
[13] Bruch, p. 254–5.
[14] Bruch, p. 251.
[15] Levenkron, p. 161.
[16] Low blood glucose or "hypoglycemia" is a more yang condition, while high blood glucose or "hyperglycemia" is a more yin condition.
[17] Bruch, p. 100 ff.
[18] Bruch, p. 90.

7. The Dietary Approach to Weight Problems and Eating Disorders ▬▬▬

The following guidelines represent the standard or average macrobiotic way of eating, and can be safely followed by anyone already experiencing generally good health to avoid the risk of health problems. At the same time, it is important to remember that no one specific dietary plan suits everyone precisely. This general pattern needs to be adjusted and freely varied to suit individual needs and circumstances. Learning how to adapt these general guidelines to suit individual needs is one of the primary purposes of macrobiotic cooking classes, which are generally available in most areas of North America, Western Europe, and in many other countries around the world.

In this chapter, the guidelines are followed by a section presenting general suggestions on how to tailor macrobiotic dietary adjustments to help balance the special conditions of overweight, underweight, anorexia nervosa, and bulimia. It is strongly recommended that these suggestions be followed under the supervision of a qualified, experienced macrobiotic teacher, and that an individual trying to reverse any of these conditions work together with the appropriate health professional or psychological counselor, as circumstances dictate.

These guidelines are presented in terms of percent of total daily volume eaten. It is not necessary to weigh or measure precisely the quantity of each food or portion; an approximate comparison of serving sizes is sufficient. (It is also unnecessary in most cases to measure calorie, protein, or carbohydrate gram content.) Whole grains can be the principal dish (at least fifty percent) at each meal, with vegetables as the primary side dish, though it is not necessary to include all side-dish categories (soups, beans, sea vegetables, etc.) at each meal. The total volume eaten will vary from person to person and from day to day, and need not be fixed; but the proper relative proportions of different food categories, regardless of total volume, are meant to be generally maintained.

WHOLE GRAINS: At least one half (fifty to sixty percent) of daily food may be cooked whole grains and their products. The majority of grains may be eaten in whole form, with a lesser amount consumed as flour, cracked grains, or otherwise processed grains. Grains may be cooked forty-five to fifty-five minutes and seasoned with a pinch of natural (unrefined) sea salt; brown rice and other whole grains are best prepared in a stainless steel or enamel and steel pressure cooker, or boiled in a pot of natural materials with a tight-fitting lid.

Grains for daily or regular use include: brown rice (short, medium, or long grain); sweet brown rice and *mochi*; barley; millet; whole oats; whole wheat berries; whole rye; whole corn; buckwheat; "pearl barley" (Job's Tears or *hato mugi*); *quinoa*; and *amaranth.*

Grain products for more occasional use include: cracked grains such as bulgar wheat, cracked wheat, cracked rye, steelcut ("Scotch") or rolled oats, corn grits or corn meal; whole grain noodles and pasta; unleavened or natural sourdough whole grain bread, traditionally prepared flat breads, tortilla, chapati, and other traditional breads; *seitan* (wheat gluten) and *fu* (puffed wheat gluten).

Fig. 11 Standard Macrobiotic Diet

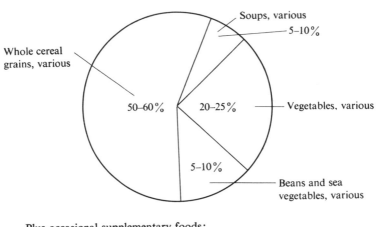

Plus occasional supplementary foods:
    Fish and seafood, using less fatty varieties
    Seasonal fruits, cooked, dried and fresh
    Nuts and seeds, various
    Natural nonaromatic and nonstimulant beverages, various
    Natural processed seasonings and condiments, various

SOUPS: One or two cups or bowls of soup (about five percent of total intake) may be consumed daily; these may contain a variety of ingredients, including seasonal vegetables, sea vegetables (particularly *kombu* or *wakame*), and occasionally grains or beans, and should be mildly seasoned with naturally processed *miso* or *tamari* soy sauce (also known as *shoyu*). Barley (*mugi*) miso and brown rice (*genmai*) miso are the most suitable for daily use.

VEGETABLES: Approximately one quarter to one third of each meal may include fresh vegetables prepared in a variety of ways, including steaming, boiling, simmering, sautéing, and others, including both dishes cooked a shorter time (from one to fifteen minutes) and with a fresher, lighter taste, and dishes cooked a longer time (from fifteen to forty-five minutes) and with a heartier taste. The proportion of these two general styles can be varied with the season and climate, the lighter, fresher dishes being more suitable for warmer conditions and the heartier, longer-cooked dishes being generally better suited to cooler conditions. In addition, up to one third of vegetable dishes may be eaten as parboiled, pressed or raw salads, and as unspiced natural pickles. *Vegetables for daily or regular use include*:

1. Root and stem vegetables: burdock, carrot, fresh and dried *daikon* (long white radish), dandelion root, lotus root (fresh and dried), onion, parsnip, radish, rutabaga, salsify, and turnip.
2. Ground vegetables: cauliflower, hard squashes (acorn, buttercup, butternut, hubbard, etc.), pumpkin and Hokkaido pumpkin.
3. Green and white leafy vegetables: broccoli, Brussel sprouts, bok choy, green cabbage, carrot tops, Chinese cabbage, chives, collard greens, daikon greens, dandelion greens, kale, leeks, mustard greens, *nappa*, parsley, scallion, turnip greens, and watercress.

Vegetables for occasional use include: celery, sweet (fresh) corn, cucumber, endive, escarole, fresh beans (string beans, snap beans, wax or yellow beans, etc.), green peas, Chinese snow peas, *jinenjo* (mountain potato), kohlrabi, lettuce, mushrooms, *shiitake* mushrooms, red cabbage, soft squashes (patty pan, summer squash, and zucchini), sprouts, and Swiss chard.

Vegetables for infrequent or rare use include: artichoke, Jerusalem artichoke or their products, bamboo shoots, beets and beet greens, docks, fennel, okra, sweet peppers (green, red, yellow, etc.), plantain, spinach, New Zealand spinach, sweet potato or yam, and taro potato.

BEANS AND SEA VEGETABLES: About five to ten percent of daily food may include cooked beans and bean products as an additional source of protein and good quality fats, and a smaller quantity of cooked sea vegetables as an additional source of minerals and vitamins. This may amount to one moderate serving of beans daily or often, and up to several tablespoons of sea vegetables daily. Beans are best well-cooked and seasoned moderately with sea salt, miso, or tamari soy sauce. Sea vegetables may be used as ingredients in other dishes (such as soups, beans, or vegetable dishes), as table condiments, and several times per week as side dishes, seasoned moderately with tamari soy sauce and/or a mild grain vinegar such as brown rice vinegar.

Beans for daily use include: *azuki* (small red) beans, brown lentils, chick-peas (garbanzo beans); soybean products such as *tofu* (fresh or dried), *tempeh*, or *natto* may also be included on a regular basis.

Beans for occasional use include: black-eyed peas, black (turtle) beans, black soybeans, great northern, kidney, lima, and navy beans, split peas, red lentils, and whole dried peas.

All edible sea vegetables are suitable for *daily or regular use*, including: agar-agar or *kanten* (as a gelatin or mold), *arame* (as a side dish), dulse, *hijiki* (as a side dish), Irish moss, kombu (for soup stocks, with beans or vegetable dishes, and as a condiment), *mekabu* (as a side dish), *nori* (as a garnish, condiment, or as a coating for rice balls or sushi), wakame (as a side dish, in soups, or as a condiment).

SUPPLEMENTARY FOODS: Seafood: Depending upon our condition and desire, a moderate volume of white-meat, non-fatty fish may be consumed up to several times per week, preferably prepared without oil (broiled, boiled, steamed, or as a soup) and served together with a larger volume of freshly steamed or boiled leafy vegetables. *Suitable varieties* include: flounder, sole, halibut, cod, schrod, haddock, trout, and others. Whole dried small fish, called *chirimen* or *chuba iriko* may be used occasionally as a seasoning or condiment.

Seeds and Nuts: A small volume of seeds may be used daily or often, either lightly roasted and lightly seasoned with sea salt or tamari and eaten as a snack, or used as condiments or in side dishes. *Suitable varieties* include: sesame, black sesame, squash, pumpkin, and sunflower seeds. Nuts may be consumed less often as they are higher in oil and more difficult to digest. Less oily nuts, including almonds, peanuts, pecans, and walnuts, may be lightly roasted, salted moderately and eaten as a snack occasionally. It is better to avoid more tropical nuts (Brazil, cashew, etc.); sesame *tahini* may be used occasionally as an ingredient in cooking, and roasted seed butters may be used occasionally as a spread.

Snacks: It is better to eat balanced meals regularly and snack infrequently, as this helps to establish a stronger condition of the digestive system. However, light snacks may be used occasionally, including: puffed whole grains, rice cakes, and popcorn; lightly roasted or toasted

107

seeds or nuts (see above); roasted grains or beans; *sushi* (rice rolled with vegetables or pickles and wrapped in nori) or rice balls; salads or pickles; and dried fruits.

Desserts: Sweet desserts may be safely enjoyed by persons in good health, usually up to three or four times per week. Unsweetened or moderately sweetened dishes of grains, sweet vegetables, and cooked or dried fruits are preferable. *Suitable ingredients* include: sweet brown rice; sweet (hard) squashes or pumpkin (other sweet vegetables such as onion, carrot, or parsnip may also be used); fresh or dried chestnuts; azuki beans; couscous; fresh or dried northern or temperate-climate fruits; nuts or seeds. *Suitable sweeteners* (when needed) include: *amazaké* (fermented sweet rice); rice syrup or barley malt syrup; dried fruits (raisins, currants, dried apples, etc.) or apple juice. *Suitable thickeners* for puddings, custards, and fillings include agar-agar (kanten) or *kuzu* starch. In general, it is best to limit or avoid the use of sweeteners on regular mealtime grain dishes, as this can interfere with good digestion. Also, the use of flour, granola toppings, crusts, and other processed grains in desserts is best kept to a minimum.

BEVERAGES: For sound digestion, it is best to avoid drinking during the course of a meal. Also, since the macrobiotic way of eating naturally contains a higher proportion of fluids in most dishes and is very low in fats and animal proteins, it is generally not necessary to drink large quantities of extra fluids as beverages. It is also better to avoid iced or very cold drinks. Normally, a moderate serving of warm or hot beverage may follow a meal, with additional drinking during the day adjusted according to thirst. It is also recommended to use unprocessed spring or deep-well water in the preparation of all teas and beverages, as well as for cooking in general.

Beverages suitable for daily or regular use include: "*bancha*" twig tea, "*bancha*" stem tea, roasted rice or roasted barley tea; boiled, spring, or well water.

Beverages for occasional use include: cereal grain coffee substitutes, roasted root beverages (dandelion, burdock, or chicory "coffees"), kombu tea, umeboshi tea, *Mu* tea, or other non-aromatic, non-stimulant teas.

Beverages for infrequent use in small amounts include: *nachi* green tea; green magma; fresh vegetable juices; temperate-climate fruit juices (apple juice or cider is preferable, especially heated); naturally processed, high quality beer or rice wine (*saké*).

COOKING SEASONINGS: In general, all seasonings may be used lightly, and not to obscure the natural taste of the ingredients used. Natural unrefined white sea salt, traditionally prepared and aged shoyu (sometimes called tamari soy sauce) and miso, and *umeboshi* (dried pickled sour plum) may all be used mildly in cooking.

High quality, mechanically expelled oils may be used, though preferably not on a daily basis, in sautéing or light pan-frying (just brushing the surface of the pan with an oil brush is best) and more infrequently for deep-frying, *tempura*, or in dressings. *Suitable varieties* include: sesame, dark or roasted sesame, squash or pumpkin, and mustard seed oils; sunflower, safflower, and olive oils may be used more infrequently; while peanut, coconut, palm, and other heavier oils may be avoided.

Additional seasonings may be used in moderation to supply various tastes, including a *sour* taste (rice or other high quality grain vinegar or umeboshi vinegar, naturally prepared sauerkraut or its juice), a *pungent* taste (fresh gingerroot, grated raw daikon or radish, chopped scallion, naturally prepared horseradish or mustard, etc.), or a sweet taste (naturally prepared *mirin* rice wine, rice or barley malt syrup).

TABLE CONDIMENTS: A variety of condiments may be used sparingly but regularly to impart additional nutrients and added flavor to various dishes. These include: baked sea vegetable powders, sea vegetable powders with crushed seeds, *gomashio* (finely ground sea salt mixed with crushed sesame seeds), ground *shiso* leaves, umeboshi plum, *tekka* (a traditional miso and root vegetable powder), *shio kombu* and *shio nori* (kombu or nori stewed with shoyu), nori flakes, and others.

A small volume of naturally pickled vegetables can also be used regularly to accompany a meal. Macrobiotic pickles are prepared from a variety of vegetables, particularly daikon and other roots, broccoli, cauliflower, and other ground vegetables, and more fibrous leafy vegetables such as kale or daikon greens, aged in sea salt, or a sea salt, shoyu, or umeboshi brine, or other salt preparation, for from several hours to over a year.

Fresh raw vegetable garnishes, such as finely chopped scallions, watercress, or parsley, may also be used regularly in small amounts to enhance the appearance, flavor, and digestibility of dishes. Grated raw daikon, ginger, or horseradish, usually seasoned with a little shoyu, are especially helpful for digestion of seafood, mochi, fried or deep-fried foods, or other slightly richer or heavier dishes.

Fig. 12   Foods to Normally Avoid for Optimum Health

Animal Products:
Red meat (beef, lamb, pork)
Poultry
Wild game
Eggs

Dairy Foods:
Milk (skim, low-fat, buttermilk, etc.)
Butter
Cheese
Yogurt
Kefir
Ice cream
Cream (sour cream, whipped cream, etc.)

Fish:
Red-meat or blue-skinned fish, such as:
Tuna
Blue fish
Swordfish
Salmon

Fats:
Lard or shortening
Margarine
Processed vegetable oils

Nuts
Brazil
Cashew
Pistachio
Hazel

Beverages:
Artificial beverages, such as:
soda, fruit-flavored beverages, colas, mixers, etc.
Alcoholic beverages
Distilled water

Processed Foods:
Instant foods
Canned foods
Frozen prepared foods
Refined (white) flour and its products
Polished (white) rice
Foods processed with:
Chemicals
Additives
Preservatives
Stabilizers
Emulsifiers
Artificial colorings, flavorings
Sprayed, dyed, or waxed foods

Stimulants:
Spices (cayenne, curry, garlic, etc.)
Commercial vinegars
Coffee
Commercial and dyed teas
Stimulating or highly aromatic teas (mint, rose hips, etc.)
Ginseng

Sweeteners:
Sugar (white, raw, brown, turbinado)
Honey
Molasses
Corn syrup
Date sugar
Fructose
Maple syrup
Carob
Saccharine, xylitol, and other artificial ("non-nutritive") sweeters

Fruits:
Tropical and sub-tropical fruits:
bananas   figs
grapefruits   prunes

Vegetables of tropical origin:
eggplant, potato, tomato

mangoes	coconut
oranges	pineapple
papayas	kiwi
avocado	

The Way of Cooking ─────────────────────

The way in which foods are prepared has a powerful effect on their
nutritional and other properties, and has a direct impact on health. In
general, the kitchen should be kept clean, uncluttered, and orderly, so
that the cook's full attention can be given to proper cooking. Techniques
such as stirring, mixing, and vegetable cutting can be carried out with
calm and orderly motions, and vegetables may be cut so that each piece
is relatively uniform to ensure even and uniform cooking for each piece.
It is preferable for dishes to be prepared fresh daily, particularly soups
and vegetable dishes; leftovers can usually be stored at room temperature
and lightly steamed or reheated when eaten. Refrigeration of leftovers
is frequently unnecessary, except in very hot or humid weather, or in the
case of dishes that easily spoil (such as fish or very moist bean dishes).

The use of longer cooking times, more salt and salt seasonings, and
pressure, generally creates dishes with a more yang, contracting effect,
while the use of shorter cooking times, more water and other seasonings,
such as oil, vinegar, or spicy tastes, and less pressure, generally produces
more yin, expanding or relaxing effects. These two types of effects can
be varied, and may be used to balance variations in climate, season, and
personal need.

The types of stove and cookware used also affect the quality of the
dishes themselves. It is preferable to use cookware made of traditional
materials, including cast iron, stainless steel, crockware, stoneware,
ceramic, enamel, glassware, and others. Aluminum, teflon coated, and
other more artificial types of cookware are best avoided. Cooking over
gas, wood, or other natural flame is preferable to the use of electric
stoves, and microwave cooking is best avoided altogether.

The proper way of cooking is so important that the reader is strongly
urged to attend qualified courses in macrobiotic cooking and to study
independently with macrobiotic cookbooks.

The Way of Eating ─────────────────────────────

In addition to the selection and preparation of the best ingredients, the way of eating itself has a strong impact on health. In general, upsetting, noisy, hurried, or chaotic circumstances tend to disrupt digestion, and can contribute to a worsening health condition. Please try to eat only when calm, relaxed, and unrushed; also, it is best to eat only when hungry.

Proper chewing is essential for good digestion and assimilation; each mouthful can be chewed at least thirty to fifty times, or until the food is fully liquified in the mouth and well mixed with saliva. Please try to avoid sleeping for at least three hours after eating, as this causes stagnation and weakness in the intestines.

When soup is part of the meal, it may be consumed as the first dish. Among various side dishes, the more yang, saltier or heavier dishes may be eaten earlier in the meal, with lighter dishes such as salads eaten toward the end of the meal. Whole grain dishes may be eaten throughout the course of the meal. A warm or hot beverage may conclude the meal or be followed by a reasonable portion of natural, mildly sweet dessert, when this is included in the meal. Eating foods too far out of this general order can also cause smooth digestion and assimilation to be disrupted.

Before and after each meal, it is a helpful and appropriate practice to express our gratitude and appreciation (verbally or silently) to nature, the universe, or God who created the food, and to reflect on the health and happiness it is dedicated to achieving. This acknowledgement may take the form of grace, prayer, song, chanting, a moment of reflective silence, or other traditional forms. To deepen our appreciation of the existence and significance of nature and its foods, we may also briefly express our thanks to parents, grandparents, and ancestors who nourished us and whose dreams we embody, to the plants who gave their lives to nourish ours, and to the farmers, shopkeepers, cooks, and other participants who contributed their energies in making this food available to us.

Dietary Adjustments for Relieving Overweight ─────────

In most cases eating according to the guidelines above will result in one's overall metabolism becoming more balanced, together with a loss of excess weight. Most people who begin eating this way, even if not for purposes of losing weight, find excess weight disappearing automatically. In some cases, a previously overweight person may even find he or she becomes overly thin; this is generally due to the fact that the person's muscle tone was poor and the Lean Body Mass was actually impoverished, despite the appearance of excess weight due to fat and water bulk. Within a period from three to nine months, a person's weight will usually stabilize.

However, it is helpful to understand some of the properties of specific foods and cooking styles, with regard to weight. Depending upon the individual situation, it may be necessary to adjust one's diet with more precision in order to achieve a proper balance. We need to keep in mind that there are generally two basic effects we need to achieve in balancing overweight. 1) in order to balance and dissolve deposits of animal fats, salt, and animal protein, more *yin*, relaxing and dissolving effects are needed. 2) in order to balance an excess of water, expansive fats, and sugars, more *yang* effects are needed.

The following are some general guidelines designed to help individuals move in the direction of this more fine-tuned understanding.

Whole Grains: Brown rice, *barley*, and *millet* are the most stabilizing. *Barley* and *"pearl barley"* (*Job's Tears*) are particularly helpful in dissolving animal fats in the muscles and liver, as are *whole corn* dishes (dried corn as opposed to sweet corn) in dissolving animal fats in the heart and blood vessels. *Buckwheat* is more yang and will often help discharge water rapidly, however it is often a little too strong to use regularly by persons who have accumulated a lot of animal foods in their systems. *Cracked grains* have a more relaxing effect, though they impart less overall vitality. *Flour products*, especially breads and *rolled oats*, tend to be more mucus forming for the intestines, and are therefore often best limited in this case. *Sweet brown rice*, *whole oats*, and *seitan* (wheat gluten) are all more rich in protein and, in the case of sweet rice and oats, in fat. While they are not helpful in losing weight, they can be very helpful for persons who need to *gain* additional weight. They also tend to produce a warming effect.

Soups: Since the body usually needs to eliminate excessive liquid, it is often best to take less liquid in the form of soups, until weight has stabilized. However, in order to help cleanse the intestines, it is especially important to have *miso soup* once daily. Soups may be taken in very small portions, such as one or two cups daily. Particularly helpful ingredients include *daikon* radish and a little *kombu* or *wakame*. *Shiitake* mushroom also helps to dissolve fats, and may be included in miso soup often. *To gain weight*, richer soups are helpful, often including grain soups and bean soups. *Miso soup* with pieces of *mochi* in it may be taken often in this case.

Vegetables: *More fibrous leafy vegetables* such as kale, watercress, radish or turnip tops, are helpful in dissolving fats in the intestinal tract and in improving absorption and elimination, especially when lightly steamed, boiled, or water sautéed. Slowly cooked *sweet tasting round or root vegetables* such as hard squash, onion, or carrot, are helpful in stabilizing blood glucose levels and satisfying sweet cravings. Hardy *root vegetables* are helpful in strengthening eliminatory and respiratory functions. *Lotus root* (fresh or dried) or *dried daikon* cooked with *kombu* and seasoned with a little shoyu and ginger or vinegar, are helpful to eliminate water and fat. Lightly cooked fresh *daikon* is also helpful in eliminating water and fats.

It may be best to have *raw salads* more infrequently while eliminating fats, as they can weaken the intestines. However, since raw vegetables can be helpful in eliminating animal fats, it is advisable to use *raw grated daikon, chopped scallions*, and other types of raw garnishes frequently as accompaniments to dishes. In place of regular salads, *boiled* or *pressed salads* may also be taken frequently or daily. Mild sautéing with oil may be used from time to time, but it is best to minimize deep-frying, tempura, and baked-vegetable dishes until weight has normalized. It is also best to avoid cooking too many vegetables together, such as stews and elaborate combinations. Lightly, freshly, and simply cooked foods will help recover a smoother metabolism and relax the stomach.

To gain weight, dishes cooked with a small amount of good quality vegetable oil may be eaten daily. *Tempura* or *deep-frying* may also be used moderately but regularly, such as once or twice per week. In addition, more well-cooked, slowly simmered dishes, such as root-vegetable stews or sweeter vegetables cooked together with *beans* or *bean products* and seasoned with a little more sea salt, miso, or shoyu, can also be helpful.

Beans and Bean Products: For overweight, it is best to limit beans to a smaller portion than usual, until weight has normalized. The smaller beans, particularly *azuki* and *brown lentil* are preferable. *Azuki* beans, especially, are helpful in strengthening the kidneys and eliminatory functions. *Tempeh* and *tofu,* while relatively rich in easily assimilable fats and protein, tend to proceed more quickly through the digestive process than regular beans, and are easier to digest. They may be used regularly, in small amounts. *In order to gain weight,* slightly larger volumes of beans may be used more often, especially when well cooked, together with sweet tasting, rich vegetables and well seasoned with *miso* or *shoyu.* In this case, those beans listed as *"for occasional use"* can be included regularly, such as *soybeans, lima beans,* or *navy* beans. In cases of both

114

under- and overweight, frequent or regular use of *natto* can be helpful in improving intestinal function.

Sea Vegetables: Daily use of sea vegetables is very important, as the minerals of sea vegetables help with the proper elimination of excessive fats as they are being discharged from the body. Especially helpful in regulating elimination are the frequent use of various side dishes cooked together with a small amount of *kombu*, such as *dried daikon* or fresh *daikon*, *lotus root*, *azuki* beans, *nishime* style vegetables, or other dishes. *Nori* may also be used daily as a condiment, and *wakame* may be taken frequently in miso soup.

Seeds, Nuts, and Snacks: To establish a regular eating pattern and smooth rhythm of the digestive process, it is best to avoid snacking as much as possible. This would apply to cases of both overweight and underweight. However, small snacks of various types may be used from time to time. In the case of overweight, it is best to limit or avoid the use of *nuts* and all oily products.

Seafoods: It is often best to minimize the intake of animal foods, including seafoods, while strong cravings for sweets, alcohol, or other strongly yin items persist, or if there is still a strong tendency toward compulsive eating. In case of *underweight*, moderate and regular use of seafood can be helpful in recovering intestinal strength.

Desserts: People new to macrobiotics frequently postpone learning to make macrobiotic-quality desserts, letting cravings for sweets build until it is difficult to avoid satisfying them without eating sugar or commercially sweet products. It is advisable to include mildly sweetened desserts from the beginning. *Kuzu* starch is a thickener that has a strengthening, tonifying effect on the intestines and stomach, while *agar-agar* (*kanten*) has a more relaxing effect. Desserts made with *flour* are best minimized, as they tend to produce more mucus and stagnation in the digestive organs. In some cases persons may experience special problems with simple sugars (such as hypoglycemia, diabetes, *Candidiasis*, or pronounced food compulsions). In such cases, it may be best to be cautious in the use of fruit or sweet desserts. Emphasizing sweet grain and vegetable dishes, and mild use of rice syrup or barley malt syrup in cooking can be helpful in such cases.

Seasonings for Cooking: *Sea salt and salt seasonings:* While some good quality minerals are necessary to properly digest foods and to help process eliminating fats and acids, it is usually best to reduce the volume of sea salt and sea-salt seasonings to a very small amount. Since our needs change and are highly individual, it is impossible to give specific guidelines. In order to help learn to regulate salt use, the following are among various ways to judge whether we may be taking too much or too little sea salt and sea-salt seasonings:

● *Common signs of too much salt use:* excessive thirst, increased cravings for oil, sweets, or for larger volumes of food in general; cannot stop eating; feeling tight or irritable; increasing darkness under the eyes or somewhat darker urine (showing a tightening of the kidneys).

● *Common signs of too little salt use:* feeling weak or sluggish, inability to make decisions; craving hard, crunchy snack foods, salt, or animal foods; digestive weakness.

Oil: Small amounts of sesame or dark (roasted) sesame oil in cooking may be used occasionally. It is best to avoid the use of oil in dressings.
Fresh gingerroot, grated daikon radish, rice vinegar, and other macrobiotic quality seasonings may be used. It is best to avoid strong spices, such as garlic, pepper, or curry.

Beverages: It is especially important to avoid chilled or iced drinks, as well as stimulating beverages such as coffee or commercial teas. While in the process of losing weight, individual needs may vary considerably; it is best to adjust liquid intake regularly according to thirst.

Table Condiments: All macrobiotic table condiments may be used moderately, taking care not to let salt consumption increase beyond a very small amount. Good homemade *gomashio* is especially helpful in recovering a proper balance of water and minerals in the body. Macrobiotic quality *pickles* are also especially important in restoring a proper balance of intestinal flora.

Dietary Adjustments for Anorexia Nervosa and Bulimia

For Anorexia	*For Bulimia*
The general goal is to produce a more warming effect and strengthen the lower body, as well as to generally balance the metabolism and dissolve fats.	The general goal is to produce a cooling and more upwardly relaxing effect, as well as to generally balance the metabolism and dissolve fats.

WHOLE GRAINS

It is especially important to chew grains thoroughly—up to one hundred times per mouthful—to improve assimilation. Grains may normally be pressure-cooked.

Emphasize: short grain and medium grain brown rice, millet, sweet brown rice, and occasionally whole oats. Seitan and mochi may be used regularly in small amounts. Grain soups may be consumed regularly.

Limit: flour products, and breads.

It is especially important to chew grains very thoroughly—up to one hundred times per mouthful—to help improve assimilation. Grains may normally be boiled and occasionally pressure-cooked.

Emphasize: short, medium, and long grain brown rice, barley, and corn. Cracked grains may be used more often.

Limit: flour products and breads, oats (any form), seitan or mochi, sweet rice.

SOUPS

It is important to have hot or warm miso soup everyday. Soups may have a rich, but not salty taste. Especially helpful ingredients include root and sweet round vegetables, and sea vegetables. Soups containing grains, vegetables, beans, or mochi may also be used from time to time.

Soups may be very lightly seasoned; in addition to miso or shoyu, a mild sour taste can also be achieved with rice or barley vinegar, umeboshi or fresh lemon juice. Especially helpful ingredients include shiitake mushroom, leafy greens, and daikon radish.

VEGETABLES

It is important to include some type of slowly cooked, long cooked vegetable dish daily. Examples include nishime style, stews, or thicker vegetable soups. Vegetables may occasionally be sautéed with a moderate amount of oil. A small amount of vegetables pickled in miso, or rice

It is important to include some types of freshly and quickly cooked vegetables daily. Examples include lightly steamed, boiled, or water-sautéed vegetables. Overall, less long-time cooking is best; cooking with oil may be infrequent Lightly pickled vegetables, pressed and boiled salads may be included bran and sea salt are very helpful to recover intestinal flora, and may be consumed regularly.

Emphasize: root vegetables, sweet round vegetables, harder or fibrous leafy vegetables.

It is best to minimize raw salads.

daily; a small raw salad may be eaten, depending upon the season.

Emphasize: all vegetables listed as "for regular use" and "for occasional use."

Limit: fried, deep-fried, or baked vegetables.

BEANS AND BEAN PRODUCTS

It is best to begin with a fairly small portion of beans (if beans are not digested well at first, they may even be initially avoided), and to gradually increase to a normal or slightly larger proportion. Beans are preferably well-cooked and moderately seasoned with miso or shoyu as well as sea salt. Daily or regular use of natto, especially in soups, is particularly beneficial. Tofu or tempeh may be used, but only when cooked, preferably together with kombu and/or strong vegetables.

Overall, intake of beans and bean products may be limited to somewhat less than the usual amount. Light (thinner consistency) bean soups and lightly cooked tofu or tempeh dishes may be used often; these may be seasoned lightly with a sour taste, as well as a little sea salt, shoyu or miso. Daily or regular use of natto, especially as a condiment with grains, is especially helpful.

SEA VEGETABLES

Emphasize: kombu, arame, and hijiki. A small side dish of arame or hijiki, cooked together with root or sweet vegetables and/or tofu, dried tofu, or tempeh and seasoned with shoyu and several drops of sesame oil, may be eaten three to four times per week. Kombu may be used daily in various dishes. Wakame may also be included regularly in miso soup.

Emphasize: kombu, nori, arame, and wakame. A side dish of either kombu, arame, or wakame, and vegetables, seasoned with a little sour taste, sweet taste and shoyu, may be eaten three to four times per week. Nori or green nori flakes may also be used regularly or daily as a condiment.

SEEDS, NUTS, AND SNACKS

It is best overall to establish regular meal times, and to avoid snacking in between meals. Seeds and nuts may be incorporated into meals. If necessary, smaller meals may be incorporated into the daily schedule. However, it is also preferable to limit the use of too many foods that exert a drying effect on the body, including well-roasted seeds and nuts, rice cakes, popcorn, and other similar foods.

It is best to establish regular meal times, and to avoid snacking in general. If necessary, small regular snacks of dried fruits, lightly toasted seeds, lightly cooked vegetables, rice balls, or sushi (without fish) may be used to compensate for awkward schedules or to avoid overly long periods between regular meals.

SEAFOODS

It is preferable to limit the use of seafood until a normal regulation of female hormones is achieved. However, if it is desired or needed for strength, a small volume (3 to 4 ounces) of white-meat fish may be used often, especially boiled, steamed, lightly broiled, or in soup. Poultry and other animal products are best avoided unless needed as emergency measures (such as when a person is unable to eat anything else).

It is best to limit intake of animal products, including seafood, until the tendency toward compulsive eating practices is eliminated and normal health is well established.

DESSERTS

In general, the sweetness of properly cooked grains and sweet vegetables will help to establish a balanced metabolism and reduce the craving for refined sweets. Whether or not it is appropriate to include especially sweet dishes such as natural macrobiotic desserts, is a highly individual concern. Many people who are experiencing eating disorders are particularly sensitive to such dishes, and may either have strong reactions to them or find it difficult or impossible to control consumption when they are included. If such dishes pose no such special problems:

Desserts made from sweetened

As desired, dried fruits and lightly

grains and vegetables, such as sweet rice, azuki beans, squash, and others, and sweetened with grain syrups or amazaké, may be used regularly. It is best to avoid raw fruit altogether; fruit may be used from time to time, preferably cooked together with a little kuzu. Desserts prepared with flour or processed grains are best to limit or avoid.

cooked fruits may be enjoyed often, particularly cooked as a kanten with agar-agar, with or without the addition of kuzu. Desserts prepared with flour are best minimized. Small amounts of raw fruits may also be used from time to time. If it is craved, a small amount of citrus, such as several slices of orange, mandarin orange, or tangerine, may be consumed.

SEASONINGS FOR COOKING

Slightly stronger sea-salt seasonings may be used; however, care should be taken that they not be too strong, as excessive salt use can lead the person to feel tight and overreact to foods. Oils may be used in small volume but often, for cooking only and not in dressings. Macrobiotic quality pungent and sweet seasonings may be used frequently; sour tasting seasonings are best limited.

All salt and salt seasonings may be used very mildly. It is preferable to avoid the use of oil, unless you are strongly craving fats. In this case, a small amount of good quality oil may be used in sautéing. Macrobiotic quality seasonings with a sweet or sour taste may be used frequently; mildly pungent flavors, such as chopped scallions or a little grated raw daikon, may also be used. Strongly spicy tastes are best avoided.

BEVERAGES

Small amounts of hot beverage may be consumed regularly, throughout the day, depending upon individual thirst. It is important that all cold or chilled drinks are avoided; vegetable or fruit juices are also best to limit or avoid. Mildly bitter tasting teas such as dandelion root, burdock, chicory, or roasted grain and bean "coffees," and "Mu" tea, may be used from time to time.

Beverage intake may be adjusted to suit thirst. If cold beverages are craved, mildly cool twig tea or cereal grain teas may be sipped. If desired, a small amount of fresh vegetable or temperate-climate fruit juice may be taken from time to time, preferably at room temperature. ("Mu" tea is best avoided.)

TABLE CONDIMENTS

Any macrobiotic quality table condiment may be used in moderate amounts. Good homemade gomashio, sea-vegetable powders, umeboshi, shio kombu, and shio nori are especially helpful. Shio kombu may also be prepared, cooked together with slices of fresh gingerroot.

All table condiments may be used very moderately. Umeboshi, nori and green nori flakes, shiso leaves, and kombu or wakame powder are especially helpful. It is also important to use small amounts of raw vegetables as garnish regularly.

8. Towards a Hamonious Way of Life

In order to establish a firm foundation for natural health, it is essential that we recognize those factors in our lives that originally led to our suffering, so that we can seek to make the appropriate changes in our life overall. It is often said that "man does not live by bread alone," and it is quite true. Nor can weight or eating disorders be completely and permanently solved simply by changing the nature of what we eat. It is also necessary to reevaluate our everyday way of life, and provide ourselves with an embracingly positive, constructive orientation.

As we said in an earlier chapter, our natural dietary goal is that we eat in order to live our lives, not that we live in order to be able to eat. Let us examine seven general areas in which we can direct our attention towards creating a more harmonious, natural way of life.

1. Harmony in Daily Lifestyle Habits

Each and every aspect of daily living has more yin and more yang aspects. For example, we naturally balance eating with activity, more physical activities with more mental activities, and more active periods with more restive times. In seeking to establish a more harmonious metabolic pattern, it is helpful to maintain a balanced regularity within these aspects of living as well. This would include the following suggestions:

- We may eat as often as our schedule and appetite direct, but it is important not to eat beyond our natural capacity. Develop the habit of leaving the table feeling satisfied but not full at the end of each meal. It is often helpful to make a point of concluding each meal with a small cup of hot tea, to give definition to the end of each meal and to avoid the tendency to keep snacking.

- Eat with good appetite and in a relaxed, unhurried manner, chewing each bite thoroughly until it becomes liquid in the mouth. To maintain a natural pace of eating, it is helpful to put utensils down between bites. It is best not to drink while eating; drink to comfortably satisfy thirst, after or between meals.

- It is best to avoid lengthy, hot baths or showers, as they can deplete the body's minerals an d have a weakening effect. Bathe as needed, but preferably use brief showers or baths with a moderate temperature. If we feel fatigued after bathing, a small hot cup of miso soup or tamari-bancha tea will help to replenish energy.

● Include some regular physical activity each day, including activities such as scrubbing floors, cleaning windows, washing and cleaning the home, carpentry or home repairs, gardening, and others. Strive for a smooth rhythm and clear, deep breathing as you go about these tasks. In addition, some form of systematic exercise may be practiced daily. As we explained earlier, this exercise should be aerobic, that is, should be practiced for continuous periods rather than in short bursts, and bring our pulse and respiration rates to a bit above our normal daily rate. However, they need not be extremely vigorous nor place a substantial strain on our system. Examples of appropriate exercise would be light athletics, various forms of yoga or martial arts, such as *aikido* or tai chi, systematic dance forms, *Do-In*,[1] as well as long walks with smooth, deep breathing. Try to establish a practical program of exercise that can be maintained over long periods, rather than starting and stopping periodically.

● In order to clarify the direction of our life and give constructive, positive form to our everyday thoughts, it is very helpful to practice some form of regular creative expression. This may take any form we prefer; keeping a daily diary of our thoughts, reflections, dreams, and ideas is especially helpful during periods of rapid change. Any form of traditional art, music, dance, woodwork, or other creative expression will help to provide a personal outlet, and divert excessive creative energies that may have previously been channeled into eating, excessive and unproductive thinking, or various negative emotional or psychological patterns.

● For the deepest and most restful sleep, and to help establish an even metabolism and calm mind, it is advisable to retire before midnight and rise early in the morning. Please avoid eating for about three hours before sleeping (the average amount of time it takes for food to leave the stomach), and avoid drinking for thirty minutes before sleeping.

2. Reconnecting with Nature

As we have seen, the origin of weight and eating disorders is the loss of our natural sense of being connected with nature, on both the conscious and unconscious, physiological levels. In order to maintain a vital health, and to keep our sense of the origin, direction, and meaning of our lives, it is important to establish an active contact with the natural forces around us, including the air, water, sunshine, the plant world, and the electromagnetic energies of the natural environment. It is also helpful to minimize the interference and more chaotic energies caused by excessively artificial environments and environmental forces.

• Go outdoors often, lightly dressed when possible, and try to walk barefoot on the soil, grass, or beach every day. Keep large green plants in the home to enrich and freshen the oxygen content of the air, and open windows whenever possible to permit the circulation of fresh air.

• All daily living materials should be as natural as possible, as synthetic fabrics and other synthetic materials can disrupt the energies we receive directly from the environment. This is particularly important for persons seeking to recover from eating disorders. Wear cotton clothing directly next to the skin, and avoid synthetic clothing when possible. Nylons, for example, may be worn for special occasions, but may be removed afterward and not worn for many hours on a routine basis. Metallic jewelry and accessories are best kept to a minimum. Cotton sheets, towels, blankets, and pillowcases, and incandescent lighting, natural wood furnishings, and cotton or wool carpeting all contribute to a more natural environment.

• Avoid or minimize the use of electric appliances close to the body, including electric razors, hair dryers, blankets, heating pads, toothbrushes, and others. Particularly in the case of anorexia or bulimia, the use of electric hair drying devices or haircurlers is best avoided temporarily. It is also particularly advisable to use a gas or wood flame for cooking, and to avoid electric or microwave cooking devices. It is also preferable to use earthenware, glassware, cast iron, and other natural cookware, rather than teflon coated, aluminum, or electric cooking pots.

• Television, particularly color television, exerts a draining and disorienting influence on the body's natural energy. The same applies to devices such as computer display terminals, video games, X-ray machines, and other such devices. If we watch television or use a computer terminal, we can try to do so in moderation and from a reasonable distance, with frequent and ample interruptions during which we can reestablish our natural clarity and strong energy.

● To reestablish and maintain the healthy functioning of our skin, it is important to minimize the use of cosmetic products, and to altogether avoid using chemically produced body-care products. Only naturally prepared products of high quality should be used, and then in moderation only.

In addition, several external treatments can help to dissolve accumulations of fats which may be blocking our system, and to restore our natural ability to exchange energies with the environment. These are listed below. For detailed directions on how to prepare these treatments, please consult the companion volume in the *Macrobiotic Food and Cooking Series*. All of the treatments described below are perfectly safe, and may be practiced moderately without danger. To determine the most appropriate ways to apply these treatments to an individual situation, it is best to personally work with an experienced macrobiotic teacher.

Ginger Compress. Normally used to increase circulation, alleviate stiffness, or to help dissolve accumulated fats. To help alleviate eating disorders, this treatment is helpful in dissolving blockages and accumulation in the small and large intestine, and may be applied daily or often during an initial several weeks, and periodically thereafter. In the case of anorexia nervosa, it is also helpful to apply hot ginger compresses to the stomach and kidney area several times per week, or even daily at first.

Taro Potato (Albi) Plaster. Often used to help draw out the minerals and fats that make up a cyst or tumor, this plaster can be helpful in releasing dissolved mucus deposits in the intestines and lower body. A taro plaster is generally preceded by a brief ginger compress (to increase circulation in the area) and then applied and left on for several hours. In cases of anorexia or bulimia, it can be helpful to follow a ginger compress over the intestines with a taro plaster, repeating daily for several days or up to one week.

Dried Daikon Leaf Hip Bath. This hot hip bath is helpful for dissolving deep deposits of fats, protein, and mucus in the female reproductive organs, and therefore is often extremely helpful in cases of bulimia and anorexia. The hot hip bath is generally followed by a mild douche prepared from bancha tea, a pinch of sea salt, and several teaspoons of rice vinegar or lemon juice.

Ginger Bath. Prepared in essentially the same manner as a ginger compress, a hot ginger foot bath can help improve circulation and warm the body. This is especially useful in increasing energy for a person with anorexia.

Lotus Root Plaster. Like the taro plaster, this plaster is usually preceded by a brief hot ginger compress. It is especially helpful in dissolving and dislodging stubborn accumulations of hardened mucus in the sinus and nasal passages, which often accompany bulimia, and are common in other conditions as well.

Whole Body Scrub. To help dissolve accumulations of fats underneath the skin, enable to pores to become more open, and revitalize the lymph and skin's functions of circulation and elimination, we can make a daily practice of scrubbing and massaging the surface of our body with a hot, damp towel until the skin becomes red. This is especially important in the case of eating disorders and overweight, to help recover and bolster the skin's eliminating functions. In such cases it is a good idea to follow this practice each morning and each night.

3. Overcoming Cravings and Food Compulsions ——

To assist the process of overcoming various cravings or habitual reliance on different foods, it is especially important to maintain a good range of variety in our selection of foods and styles of preparation. In making a transition to a more moderate way of eating, people often experience times when the taste, texture, or other qualities of previous foods suddenly become strongly attractive, leading to the desire to "binge" on some of those foods. These occurrences also often give rise to feelings of guilt and self-recrimination, and may become part of habitual and complex thought patterns. One may begin to think things such as, "I knew I couldn't change, now I've confirmed it," or, "I'm doomed to fail at this, I might as well give up," and so forth.

Strive to put aside these dualistic reactions; everyone is human, and there are reasons why these things occur. Don't let these occasions, if they arise, escalate into elaborate internal dialogues; accept them, and let them go. Actually, we can use such occasions as opportunities for learning more about ourselves, and about yin and yang. Reflecting upon such experiences, we often discover that our macrobiotic practice has been overly restrictive or one-sided, for example, using only lightly steamed vegetable dishes with nothing well-cooked, or vice versa. These experiences can be educational and lead to improved finesse and creativity in cooking.

At the same time, it is equally important to get control of such situations before they do escalate and lead us back into extreme eating patterns. One helpful point is to strive to maintain our new sense of respect for food, chewing slowly and eating with a sense of gratitude, even if we are eating foods we had not planned to be eating. And, if cravings for specific foods do arise, it is often helpful to consume moderate amounts of high quality foods having the similar taste, texture, or other property of the food craved. The Figure below provides some examples of how this principle can be applied.

It is also helpful to remember that the overuse of sea salt and salt seasonings can lead to intensified cravings. Conversely, the complete elimination of salt from the diet will also often lead to strong cravings.

Fig. 13   Substitution Examples When Craving Extreme Foods

Craving	Transitional Food	Ideal
Meat	fish, seafood	well-cooked *seitan*, *tempeh*, *tofu* beans
Eggs, dairy foods, fatty or greasy foods	fried or deep-fried grains, beans, bean products; nuts, nut butters, soy milk	soy products: *tempeh*, *tofu*, *natto*; roasted seeds
Tropical fruits & juices, artificial beverages, cold drinks	organic temperate-climate fruits, juices	organic temperate-climate fruits (dried or cooked) and juices in small volume and in season
Sugar, sweets	honey, maple syrup	cooked or dried fruits, natural grain sweeteners
Strong alcohol	high-quality beer, *saké* (rice wine) in small volume	fermented grain, bean and vegetables foods: *tempeh*, sauerkraut, fresh pickles, *amazake*, *miso*, etc.
Coffee, black tea, soft drinks, diet drinks	herb teas, green tea, mineral water	*bancha* twig tea, grain coffees, root coffees

4.   A Balanced Mind and Emotions ────────

The decision to eat in a different way is more than a choice of different fuels. When we choose a new way of eating, whether consciously or unconsciously, we are choosing a new way of being. Keep in mind, though, that it takes some time for old habits to dissolve and new ways of living to be firmly established. The change from sickness to health, or from imbalance to balance, rarely proceeds in a straight line. Individuals will likely experience transient periods of feeling worse, alternating with times of more clear cut improvement when they are feeling much better.

Our weight and sense of control or clarity over our eating patterns are liable to follow the same course. Most people experience periods when they feel they are "slipping back." This is actually a naturally occurring cycle—an example of the universal rhythms of yin and yang which exists everywhere. During any more difficult periods, it is helpful to read the personal accounts of those whose lives have changed through adopting macrobiotics, such as the experiences recounted in the variety of such books now available. It is also helpful to renew, strengthen, and clarify our contact with nature, and to keep up an active exchange with family and friends, rather than isolating ourself.

Remember that the *quality* of body weight needs to change as well as the actual number of pounds. Since muscle actually weighs much more than fat, it is not unusual to go through a period when we replace a great deal of body fat with an amount of newly toned muscle, without any of this positive change being reflected in our bathroom scales. Because of this, it is best to avoid using our actual body weight as *the* measure of our progress and change. The clarity of our thinking and overall sense of positive direction in our life are far better indicators.

We suggest that individuals seek to live each day happily, without being preoccupied with their condition or with their food, or dwelling on negative thoughts or emotions. If such negative feelings or images do arise, it is not necessary to feel guilty or defeated because of their presence. Often, when we are more actively dissolving and discharging deposits of stored excesses from the body, we temporarily experience the feelings and emotions that accompanied those physical excesses at the time we were originally eating them. It is not unusual for such "emotional discharge" to take the form of unusual dreams or sudden passing moods. Rather than reattaching to these feelings, consider them as excesses that are being expelled, which will lead to a more peaceful condition. By observing the more yin or more yang nature of such transient feelings, we may be able to identify what sorts of excesses they

128

represent. Some examples are listed below. As we become familiar with using yin and yang as a way of observing and understanding life, we will find other examples.

Fig. 14   Examples of Excessively Yin and Yang Emotional States

More Yang	More Yin
aggressive, angry	defensive, negative
over-confident	under-confident
self-asserting	self-denying
overly concerned with the past	overly concerned with the future
denial of spiritual or philosophical affairs	denial of material or practical affairs
blaming, accusing	worrying, complaining
feel like shouting	feel like crying

5. Balancing Our Self Image Through Self Reflection

Our state of health and physical condition are a direct reflection of our way of viewing ourself. Sickness results not only from poor choices in daily food and drink, but also from the way of education, training, and individual thinking that creates those choices. This generally includes an unhappy or imbalanced self image. Living in the modern technological, fast-paced world, nourished on a diet and societal orientation that is drastically apart from nature, it is easy to come to see ourselves as separate, lone beings, fighting for survival in an essentially hostile world.

This fragmented view often leads to a kind of split image of ourselves. On the one hand, we may see ourselves as being inferior, tiny, and insignificant. On the other hand, we may sometimes feel we are the most important thing in the world, thinking, 'if I don't take this kind of attitude, who will watch out for me?'

This kind of thinking plays havoc with our natural sense of self-esteem, as it makes us both under-important and over-important at the same time. By adopting a simpler, more embracing perspective, we begin to see that we are not at all separate. We are manifestations of the natural world that has created us and constantly nourishes us with air, sunlight, and food. As we begin to sense our direct kinship with our environment, we naturally come to see that we are no more important, and no less important, than any other of nature's creations.

Once we realize that we are part of life's continuous fabric, we begin to realize that all the influences in our daily lives, even apparent failures or difficulties, are serving to support us and challenge us to clarify our direction and strengthen our own capabilities. By appreciating life in all its dimensions, we increase our faith in the integrity of the universe, and life increasingly becomes a joyful and amusing adventure.

This process is all contained within the art of self reflection. As a daily practice to develop and deepen this sort of awareness, self reflection may include simple forms of quiet prayer or meditation. An essential part of our contemplation is that we avoid thinking in elaborate or complicated ways. Questions we might ask and areas wherein we might seek guidance may include the following:

Seven Daily Self Reflections

1. Did I eat in harmony with my environment, my history, and my purpose in life?

2. Did I think of my parents, relatives, friends, teachers, and elders with love and respect?

3. Did I happily greet everyone I met today and express an interest in their lives?

4. Did I contemplate the sky, trees, plants, and stars, and marvel at the wonders of nature?

5. Did I contemplate the works of art, culture, industry, and human endeavor and ingenuity, and marvel at the aspirations of human society?

6. Did I thank everyone and appreciate everything I experienced today?

7. Did I carry out my activities today with faith and commitment, and thereby contribute to the dream of a more peaceful world?

6. Harmony in Relations with Family, Friends, and Society

As our sense of self grows clearer, this will naturally extend itself to our everyday relationships with others in our life. Even in cases where one person eats macrobiotically and other family members or friends continue to eat and live in a way that may harm their health or make them unhappy, a deeper sense of unity and harmony can be created by our exercising a more peaceful and gracious expression. Helpful daily practices in this area would include:

● Greet everyone you meet happily and with appreciation.

● Initiate and maintain an active, regular correspondence with all family members, often expressing your gratitude for their part in your life.

● Enlarge your circle of friends and acquaintances, including people from all walks of life.

● Share your food often with others. Food taken in company is always more satisfying, and the act of sharing good food has always been a universal expression of human communion.

● Put aside some time daily to make yourself quiet and peaceful, and offer your thanks to your ancestors, teachers, and elders, and your dedication to help and support those who will look to you for guidance. This may take the form of a simple meditation or prayer, or a simple daily dedication towards the furthering of human peace and happiness.

7. Harmony with Our Life Purpose ────────────

Though it is often personal health concerns that lead people to learn about macrobiotics, the decision to eat macrobiotically carries a far broader meaning in today's troubled world. The act of choosing unrefined whole foods, for example, even when personal health is the sole conscious criterion, also makes a strong economic and ecological statement.

Some people experience this fact as a conflict, and eventually feel pressed to abandon their new dietary ways because they do not conform to society's existing way of eating and overall values. In order to fully incorporate the macrobiotic approach into our life, and fully experience its benefits, it is often necessary to consciously face, transform, and overcome this sense of conflict.

First, it is important to realize that while eating macrobiotically often poses new social challenges, such as when eating out or at gatherings of friends, this situation is rapidly changing. As the emerging dietary common sense gradually establishes itself, it is becoming progressively easier

to harmonize our macrobiotic dietary values with the rest of society.
Further, it is essential to realize that the values this way of eating
challenges are precisely those that our civilization needs to change, if we
are to avoid further suffering and the possibility of disastrous events.
The modern approaches to consumption, overuse of technology, divorce
from nature, and behavioral extremes, are the root cause of the eating
disorders we are striving to overcome. They are likewise the root cause
of much of our broader social difficulties.

Simply being alive at the present time poses unique challenges, and
offers historically unprecedented opportunities for positive change on
a massive scale. Rather than retreating from these challenges to our
survival, the decision to eat macrobiotically and to embrace the harmonious, unifying perspective underlying this approach, can enable us to
open the door to these historical opportunities and contribute to the
realization of world health and world peace.

---

[1] Please refer to the author's *Book of Do-In* for a variety of exercises.

Resources

Macrobiotics International in Boston and its major educational centers in the United States, Canada, and around the world offer ongoing classes for the general public in macrobiotic cooking and traditional food preparation and natural processing. They also offer instruction in Oriental medicine, shiatsu massage, pregnancy and natural child care, yoga, meditation, science, culture and the arts, and world peace and world government activities. Macrobiotics International Educational Centers also provide way of life guidance services with trained and certified consultants, make referrals to professional health care associates, and cooperate in research and food programs in hospitals, medical schools, prisons, drug rehabilitation clinics, nursing homes, and other institutions. In scores of other cities and communities, there are smaller Macrobiotics International learning centers, residential centers, and information centers offering some classes and services.

Most of the foods mentioned in this book are available at natural food stores, selected health food stores, and a growing number of supermarkets around the world. Macrobiotic specialty items are also available by mail order from various distributors and retailers.

Please contact Macrobiotics International in Boston or other national centers listed below for information on regional and local activities in your area, as well as whole foods outlets and mail order sources.

Global Headquarters
Macrobiotics International
Box 568
Brookline, Mass. 02147
617–738–0045

Australia
Australian Macrobiotic
  Association
1 Carlton St., Prahran
Melbourne, 3181
Australia
03–529–1620

Belgium
Oost West Centrum
  Kushi Institute
Consciencestraat 48
Antwerpen, 2000
Belgium
03–230–13–82

Bermuda
Macrobiotic Center
  of Bermuda
In-The-Lee, Deepwood
  Drive Fairyland
Pembroke, Bermuda
809–29–5–2275

Britain
Community Health
  Foundation
188–194 Old Street
London, ECIV 9BP
England
01–251–4076

Canada
861 Queen Street
Toronto, Ontario
M6J IC4, Canada

France
Le Grain Sauvage
  Macrobiotic
  Association
15 Rue Letellier, 75015
Paris, France
33–1–828–4773

134

Germany
Ost West Zentrum
Eppendorfer
 Marktplatz
13 D-2000, Hamburg 20
040-47-27-50

Holland
Oost West Centrum
 Kushi Institute
Achtergracht 17
1017 WL Amsterdam
Holland
020-240-203

Hong Kong
Conduit RD 41A
Rome CT. 8D Hong
 Kong, Hong Kong
5-495-268

Israel
24 Amos Street
Tel Aviv, Israel
442979

Italy
Fondazione Est Ovest
Via de'Serragli 4
50124 Florence, Italy

Japan
Macrobiotics—Tokyo
20-9 Higashi Mine
Ota-ku, Tokyo 146
Japan
03-753-9216

Lebanon
Mary Naccour
Couvent St. Elie
Box 323 Antelias
Beirut, Lebanon

Norway
East West Center
Frydenlundsgt 2 0169
Oslo 1, Norway
02-60-47-79

Portugal
Unimave
Rua Mouzinha da
 Silveira 25, 1200
Lisbon, Portugal
1-557-362

Switzerland
Ost West Zentrum
Postfach 2502, Bern
3001 Switzerland
031-25-65-40

United Arab Emirates
Box 4943 SATWA
Dubai, United Arab
 Emirates
040440-031
 (national)
97-1-44-4-0031
 (international)

United Nations
United Nations
 Macrobiotics Society
c/o Katsuhide Kitatani
U.N. Development
 Programme
1 United Nations
Plaza, New York
N. Y. 10017
212-906-5844

United States
Kushi Institute
17 Station Street
Brookline, Mass.
02147
617-738-0045

Bibliography

Macrobiotic Health Education Series

Kushi, Michio. *A Natural Approach: Allergies.* Edited by Mark Mead and John D. Mann. Tokyo: Japan Publications, Inc., 1985.
———. *A Natural Approach: Diabetes and Hypoglycemia.* Edited by John D. Mann. Tokyo: Japan Publications, Inc., 1985.

Macrobiotic Food and Cooking Series

Kushi, Aveline. *Cooking for Health: Allergies.* Edited by Rosalind Rhodes. Tokyo: Japan Publications, Inc., 1985.
———. *Cooking for Health: Diabetes and Hypoglycemia.* Edited by Rosalind Rhodes. Tokyo: Japan Publications, Inc., 1985.

Cookbooks

Aihara, Cornellia. *Macrobiotic Kitchen.* Tokyo: Japan Publications, Inc., 1983.
———. *The Do of Cooking,* Chico. Calif.: George Ohsawa Macrobiotic Foundation, 1972.
Esko, Edward and Wendy. *Macrobiotic Cooking for Everyone.* Tokyo: Japan Publications, Inc., 1980.
Esko, Wendy. *Introducing Macrobiotic Cooking.* Tokyo: Japan Publications, Inc., 1978.
Estella, Mary. *Natural Foods Cookbook: Vegetarian Dairy-free Cuisine.* Tokyo: Japan Publications, Inc., 1985.
Kushi, Aveline. *How to Cook with Miso.* Tokyo: Japan Publications, Inc., 1978.
Kushi, Aveline, with Alex Jack. *Aveline Kushi's Complete Guide to Macrobiotic Cooking for Health, Harmony, and Peace.* N. Y.: Warner Publishing Co., 1984.
Kushi, Aveline, with Wendy Esko. *The Changing Seasons Macrobiotic Cookbook.* Wayne, N. J.: Avery Publishing Group, 1984.
Ohsawa, Lima. *Macrobiotic Cuisine.* Tokyo: Japan Publications, Inc., 1984.

Other Macrobiotic or Related Books

Aihara, Herman. *Basic Macrobiotics.* Tokyo: Japan Publications, Inc., 1985.
Brown, Virginia, with Susan Stayman. *Macrobiotic Miracle: How a Vermont Family Overcame Cancer.* Tokyo: Japan Publications, Inc., 1985.
Dufty, William. *Sugar Blues.* New York: Warner, 1975.
Heidenry, Carolyn. *An Introduction to Macrobiotics: A Beginner's Guide to the Natural Way of Health.* Brookline Mass.: Aladdin Press, 1984.
———. *Making the Transition to a Macrobiotic Diet.* Brookline, Mass.: Aladdin Press, 1984.
Ineson, Rev. John. *The Way of Life: Macrobiotics and the Spirit of Chris-*

136

tianity. Tokyo: Japan Publications, Inc., 1985.

Kohler, Jean and Mary Alice. *Healing Miracles from Macrobiotics.* West Nyack, N.Y.: Parker, 1979.

Kotzsch, Ronald E. *Macrobiotics: Yesterday and Today.* Tokyo: Japan Publications, Inc., 1985.

Kushi, Aveline. *Lessons of Day and Night.* Wayne, N. J.: Avery Publishing Group, 1984.

Kushi, Michio. *The Book of Dō-In: Exercise for Physical and Spiritual Development.* Tokyo: Japan Publications, Inc., 1979.

Kushi, Michio. *The Book of Macrobiotics* (Revised edition), Tokyo: Japan Publications, Inc., 1987.

————. *Cancer and Heart Disease: The Macrobiotic Approach to Degenerative Disorders* (Revised edition), Tokyo: Japan Publications, Inc., 1985.

————. *The Era of Humanity.* Edited by Sherman Goldman. Brookline, Mass.: East West Journal, 1980.

————. *How to See Your Health: The Book of Oriental Diagnosis.* Tokyo: Japan Publications, Inc., 1980.

————. *Macrobiotic Home Remedies.* Edited by Marc Van Cauwenberghe. Tokyo: Japan Publications, Inc., 1985.

————. *Natural Healing through Macrobiotics.* Tokyo: Japan Publications, Inc., 1987.

————. *Your Face Never Lies.* Wayne, N.J.: Avery Publishing Group, 1983.

Kushi, Michio and Aveline. *Macrobiotic Pregnancy and Care of the Newborn.* Tokyo: Japan Publications, Inc., 1984.

————. *Macrobiotic Child Care & Family Health.* Tokyo: Japan Publications, Inc., 1986.

Kushi, Michio, with Alex Jack. *The Cancer Prevention Diet.* N. Y.: St. Martin's Press, 1983.

————. *Diet for a Strong Heart: Michio Kushi's Macrobiotic Dietary Guidelines for the Prevention of High Blood Pressure, Heart Attack, and Stroke.* New York: St. Martin's Press, 1985.

Kushi, Michio and the East West Foundation. *Cancer and Heart Disease: The Macrobiotic Approach to Degenerative Disorders.* Edited by Edward Esko. Tokyo: Japan Publications, Inc., 1982.

Mendelsohn, Robert, S. *Confessions of a Medical Heretic.* Chicago: Contemporary Books, 1979.

————. *Male Practice.* Chicago: Contemporary Books, 1980.

Nussbaum, Elaine, *Recovery: From Cancer to Health Through Macrobiotics.* Tokyo: Japan Publications, Inc., 1985.

Ohsawa, George. *Cancer and the Philosophy of the Far East.* Oroville, Calif.: George Ohsawa Macrobiotic Foundation, 1971.

Ohsawa, George, with William, Dufty. *You Are All Sanpaku.* N. Y.: University Books, 1965.

Sattilaro, Anthony, with Tom Monte. *Recalled by Life: The Story of My Recovery from Cancer.* Boston: Houghton-Mifflin, 1982.

Tara, William. *Macrobiotics and Human Behavior.* Tokyo: Japan Publications, Inc., 1985.

Index